INTERMITTENT FASTING FOR WOMEN OVER 60

The Ultimate Guide on how to quickly and easily reset stubborn weight, boost metabolism, and maintain a healthy lifestyle with intermittent fasting

By

LISA BROWN

All rights reserved. No part of this publication may be reproduced or transmitted in any form or by any means, including photocopying, recording, or other electronic or mechanical methods, without the prior written permission of the publisher, except in the case of brief quotations embodied in critical reviews and certain other noncommercial use permitted by copyright law.

Copyright © Lisa Brown, 2022.

Table of Content

Copyright page

Introduction

Chapter 1: What Is Intermittent Fasting?

- How does intermittent fasting function?
- Can everyone practice Intermittent Fasting?
- Potential health benefits of Intermittent Fasting
- The advantages and disadvantages of intermittent fasting

Chapter 2: Types of Intermittent Fasting

Chapter 3: How to Start Intermittent Fasting and Stick With It

Chapter 4: How to Manage Weight Loss With Intermittent Fasting For People Over 60

Chapter 5: Foods to Eat and avoid on an Intermittent Fasting Diet

- Things to Know When Combining Intermittent Fasting with Particular Diets
- How to safely fast and shorten your fasting period

Chapter 6: Working out during your intermittent fasting

Chapter 7: Recipes for intermittent fasting

Conclusion

Introduction

Women of today, especially women over 60 are tremendously motivated to become and maintain their health. Additionally, there are a few wonderful ways to spend your golden years now that people are living into their 90s. Others spend their days at a vacation home in the mountains, while some purchase an RV and cruise the country. Relaxing and having fun are the main goals of retirement. But if you're sick and miserable a lot of the time, you can't enjoy your time. The answer is frequently Intermittent Fasting for women over 60.

Intermittent fasting has grown in popularity among women over 60 for a variety of reasons, including this. Intermittent fasting is a useful strategy for helping you feel powerful and healthy. But there are a few things you must be aware of. It's more crucial than ever to see your doctor before beginning a new fasting program as you become older. If you want to know if beginning a diet is a suitable option for someone your age and in your health, consult your doctor.

A sequence of hormonal changes known as menopause is coming to an end for the majority of women over 60. These modifications, together with the natural aging process, have been shown to increase belly obesity, osteoporosis, more rapid muscle loss, and other problematic conditions.

According to research, fasting can enhance your metabolism, and mental health, and possibly even prevent some malignancies. It can also prevent muscle, nerve, and joint conditions that can afflict women over 60.

For women over 60, intermittent fasting may aid in weight loss and lower the risk of developing common ailments associated with aging. A recent study found that intermittent fasting can lower blood pressure. The research shows that altering the gut flora while fasting decreases blood pressure.

For many women over 60, losing weight is a major issue in addition to trying to enhance their health. Reduced muscle mass, an aching body, a slower metabolism, and sleep problems are just a few factors that make losing weight more difficult after the age of 60. The chance of developing serious health conditions including diabetes, heart attacks, and cancer can be significantly decreased by decreasing fat, especially unhealthy belly fat.

Of course, the likelihood of contracting numerous diseases rises with age. When it comes to weight loss and lowering the risk of acquiring common age-related ailments, intermittent fasting for women over 60 may in certain situations act as a veritable fountain of youth.

It might be difficult to lose weight and get healthier at any age, but it becomes much more difficult after the age of 60. Many different things can cause this. Often, slow metabolism is a real culprit. Your metabolism increases with your level of lean muscle. But as we age, lean muscle mass declines and we frequently become less active than before. What happened?

Intractable body fat that just won't seem to go away.

Weight gain of some kind is unavoidable given all the changes that take place in our bodies. At the very least, we have excess weight around our midsection, making it difficult to maintain a healthy lifestyle every day.

Therefore, the idea of intermittent fasting beyond 60 is a possibility for weight loss. Perhaps you've heard of this kind of eating window strategy as a means of shedding pounds and enhancing your health, but you're not sure if it's suited for you. You have my full support, my friend.

Being a seasoned grazer and lover of breakfast in the morning, the idea of going without food for a certain amount of time is a little intimidating. I then decided to learn more about this intermittent eating pattern by conducting some studies.

Women over 60 can lose weight and improve their health with intermittent fasting, but it's crucial to discover the ideal plan that works for you. Changing your eating habits can help you achieve your goals without having any unwanted side effects if you go about it the proper way.

Intermittent fasting might be the best option if you're just beginning your weight loss journey or if you've been working hard to eat healthily and need a new method.

Chapter 1

What Is Intermittent Fasting?

Intermittent fasting is a scheduled strategy for eating, not a diet. While many diets concentrate on what you should eat, intermittent fasting is all about when you should eat.

Contrary to many other diet regimens, intermittent fasting does not list specific foods that should be consumed or avoided. Intermittent fasting may be good for your health and help you lose weight, hence, it's not for everyone.

Alternating between eating and fasting times is known as intermittent fasting. To eat only for a brief period each day or to alternate between eating days and not eating days may be challenging for some people at first.

People frequently employ intermittent fasting too:

- To make life simpler
- weight loss,
- Better general health, and
- Reduce the negative impacts of aging, for example, to improve their general health and wellbeing.

Even though most healthy, well-nourished persons can safely fast, people with medical issues may not choose to do so.

Our bodies have evolved to be able to survive for several hours, or perhaps several days, or longer, without eating. Before humans learned how to farm, they were hunters and gatherers in the prehistoric era. They evolved to survive — and thrive — for extended periods without food. Having to: The time and effort required to hunt game and collect nuts and berries was considerable.

Maintaining a healthy weight was simpler even fifty years ago. At that time, there were no computers and TV shows ended at 11 p.m. People stopped eating because they went to bed. They were substantially smaller in size. In general, more individuals worked and played outside and engaged in more physical activity.

TV, the internet, and other forms of entertainment are readily available right now. We stay up later to watch our favorite programs, play games and participate in online discussions. and gatherers who developed to survive — and thrive — for extended periods without food. To watch our favorite shows, play games, and chat online, we stay up late. We spend most of the day and night lounging around and munching.

A higher risk of obesity, type 2 diabetes, heart disease, and other ailments can result from eating more calories and being less active. According to scientific research, intermittent fasting might be able to buck these tendencies.

In this way, it's not a diet in the traditional sense; rather, it's more appropriately referred to as an eating pattern.

Daily fasts of 16 hours or twice-weekly 24-hour fasts are common intermittent fasting techniques.

Throughout all of human evolution, people have observed fasts. The ancestors of modern hunter-gatherers did not have supermarkets, refrigerators, or year-round access to food. They occasionally struggled to find food.

Because of this, humans have evolved to be able to go for extended periods without eating.

In actuality, fasting occasionally is more natural than consistently eating 3–4 (or more) meals each day.

In religions including Islam, Christianity, Judaism, and Buddhism, fasting is also frequently practiced for spiritual or religious purposes.

How does intermittent fasting function?

There are many various approaches to intermittent fasting, but they all begin with deciding on a regular eating and fasting window of time. You may, for instance, experiment with only eating for eight hours each day and fasting the other sixteen. Alternatively, you might decide to just eat one meal per day on alternate days of the week. There are numerous different intermittent fasting plans.

The body uses up all of its sugar reserves and begins to burn fat after some time without meals. I call this metabolic switching.

Intermittent fasting contrasts with the typical eating habit of most Americans, who eat during their waking hours. If a person is eating three meals a day plus snacks and isn't exercising, they are constantly consuming calories and aren't burning off their fat reserves.

The way intermittent fasting works is by extending the time it takes for your body to finish burning the calories from your last meal and start burning fat.

Can everyone practice Intermittent Fasting?

Intermittent fasting is not advised if you take any medications, are pregnant, attempting to get pregnant, are nursing a baby, are pregnant, have a chronic health condition, or are any of the above.

People in the following groups should exercise extra caution, in my opinion:

- If you've experienced eating issues in the past,
- Having a low BMI or being underweight
- If hypoglycemia attacks are common for you (low blood sugar)

- if you are currently using any prescription drugs, particularly ones that reduce blood sugar
- If you have chronic stress or sleeplessness
- If you're attempting to conceive, pregnant, or nursing
- When experiencing amenorrhea (absent or irregular periods)

Adolescence is a crucial time for growth, so whether you are a teen or a young adult, take advantage of it.

If you fit into any of these categories, you can ask your doctor if intermittent fasting might be appropriate for your situation under their supervision, but you'll probably need close supervision.

Potential health benefits of Intermittent Fasting

An eating habit is known as intermittent fasting cycles between eating and fasting times.

Intermittent fasting comes in numerous forms, including the 16/8 and 5:2 schedules.

Many studies have shown that it can have significant advantages for your body and brain.

Here are health benefits of intermittent fasting:

1. Modifies how hormones, cells, and genes function

The body goes through several changes when you go without food for a period.

For instance, your body starts vital cellular repair procedures and modifies hormone levels to make body fat that has been accumulated more accessible.

Here are a few alterations that take place in your body while you're fasting:

- **Glucose levels:** Significant drops in blood insulin levels facilitate fat burning.

- **Levels of Human Growth Hormones (HGH):** Human growth hormone (HGH) levels in the blood could rise sharply. Increased levels of this hormone promote muscular growth and fat loss, among many other advantages.

- **Cell regeneration:** The body initiates crucial cellular repair activities, such as clearing cells of trash.

- **Expression of genes:** Several genes and substances involved in aging and disease prevention have undergone advantageous modifications. These alterations in hormone levels, cellular processes, and gene expression are linked to many of the advantages of intermittent fasting. Human growth hormone (HGH) levels rise and insulin levels fall while fasting. Additionally, your cells start crucial cellular repair procedures and modify which genes they express.

2. Can aid in weight loss and visceral fat reduction

It is well-recognized that controlling your intake has a significantly higher influence on weight loss than deciding how often or when to eat. But intermittent fasting can help you keep a calorie deficit that leads to weight loss.

Just because you are intermittent fasting does not mean you are automatically in a calorie deficit. Some people still struggle to stay within a healthy calorie range, despite limiting the amount of time they spend eating.

It has been demonstrated that calorie restriction can reduce body weight and visceral fat, however maintaining a healthy caloric deficit over an extended length of time can be challenging. Given that recent human studies have shown considerable reductions in body weight and visceral fat, intermittent fasting is regarded as a helpful method to enhance weight loss.

It can be challenging to encourage people to cut back on their eating while also fasting, and variables like protein consumption, length of fasting, and food quality can affect the results of long-term studies of intermittent fasting. It is unknown if yo-yo dieting or weight gain is likely to happen when fasting is discontinued, so more research is required to evaluate any long-term weight loss benefits of intermittent fasting.

It's possible that intermittent fasting causes weight loss for reasons more than merely calorie restriction. More weight loss may result from fasting's physiological changes than from calorie restriction alone, such as lower levels of insulin and the hormone leptin.

In general, intermittent fasting will cause you to eat fewer meals.

You will consume fewer calories unless you make up for it by eating significantly more at the other meals.

3. Intermittent fasting also improves hormone activity to aid in weight loss.

Increased concentrations of norepinephrine (noradrenaline), lower insulin levels, and higher HGH levels all promote the breakdown of body fat and make it easier to utilize it as fuel.

Because of this, short-term fasting helps you burn more calories by raising your metabolic rate.

Intermittent fasting, therefore, affects both sides of the calorie equation. It improves calorie expenditure (metabolic rate) while decreasing food intake (reduces calories).

You can eat fewer calories while also modestly improving your metabolism by engaging in intermittent fasting. It is a highly powerful strategy for shedding pounds and visceral fat.

At the end of the day, maintaining sustainable weight loss involves more than just controlling our calorie intake with techniques like intermittent fasting. Our capacity to reduce stress, maintain a healthy weight, get enough sleep, and lead an active lifestyle are all influencing variables.

4. May lessen the risk of cancer

Uncontrolled cell development is a feature of cancer.

There have been various positive benefits of fasting on metabolism that may lower the risk of developing cancer.

Additionally, some studies indicate that those who fasted experienced fewer negative effects from chemotherapy.

In research on both animals and humans, intermittent fasting has been proven to aid in the prevention of cancer. It can help lessen the negative effects of chemotherapy, according to human research.

5. Enhances brain function

Oftentimes, what is beneficial for the body is also good for the brain.

Various metabolic processes that are known to be crucial for brain health are improved by intermittent fasting.

Intermittent fasting lessens:

- Inflammation brought caused by oxidative damage
- Blood sugar levels
- Insulin resistance

Studies on mice and rats have suggested that intermittent fasting may promote the creation of new nerve cells, which should be advantageous for brain health.

Additionally, fasting raises levels of the brain hormone known as a brain-derived neurotrophic factor (BDNF). Depression and many other issues with the brain have been linked to a BDNF shortage.

Additionally, research on animals has demonstrated that intermittent fasting guards against stroke-related brain damage.

The health of the brain may be significantly improved by intermittent fasting. It might promote the development of new neurons and shield the brain from harm.

6. Enhances Insulin Resistance, Which Can Aid in the Management and Prevention of Diabetes

By decreasing leptin concentrations—a hormone produced by fat cells to control hunger—and raising adiponectin, a hormone involved in glucose and lipid metabolism, intermittent fasting and weight loss may help lower fasting blood glucose and enhance insulin sensitivity.

People who intermittently fasted had lower blood glucose levels in studies where fasting was employed as a weight-loss intervention and method for maintaining a healthy weight, which also happens to be a key objective in the prevention and treatment of diabetes.

Although studies indicate that intermittent fasting generally has a good impact on blood sugar levels, these potential advantages may be largely driven by weight loss and body fat percentage reductions brought on by caloric restriction.

Both people with and without diabetes may benefit from intermittent fasting to enhance glycemic control and reduce insulin resistance while losing weight.

7. Might Aid in Cholesterol Reduction

When eating a nutritious diet throughout your non-fasting times, your cholesterol may also decrease following intermittent fasting.

Intermittent fasting has been associated with improved lipid profiles, including decreased total cholesterol, LDL (low-density lipoprotein), and triglyceride levels in healthy and obese people.

If you're worried about having high cholesterol, try embracing healthy lifestyle practices like regular exercise and a diet high in high-fiber, low-saturated fat foods.

8. Encourages Heart Wellness

Based on findings from primarily animal studies, intermittent fasting may protect our hearts by avoiding heart disease and promoting recovery after heart attacks.

Intermittent fasting has been shown to reduce risk factors for heart disease in human trials, including:

- Lower blood pressure
- Reducing lipid and cholesterol levels in the blood
- Lowering C-reactive proteins and cytokines, which are inflammatory agents, and
- Normalising blood glucose levels

Your resting heart rate could be decreased as a result of the calorie reduction and metabolic changes brought on by intermittent fasting (HR). varyingly increase your heart rate, and enhance vasodilation and blood flow.

Even while fasting could have certain health benefits, improving our food and lifestyle might help us develop wholesome habits that will promote our well-being.

10. Aids in the maintenance and function of the brain

By guarding neurons in the brain against degradation and dysfunction, intermittent fasting may maintain brain health and function, enhance memory and mental performance, and boost brain health.

In neurological conditions like epilepsy, Alzheimer's, Parkinson's, and stroke, intermittent fasting may be a helpful treatment.

It's important to keep in mind that these possible advantages may result from more than just the act of fasting; optimal blood sugar levels, lower inflammation, and decreased body fat have all been related to good brain performance.

11. Keeps Cells Young and Healthy

When we fast, we offer our body the chance to recharge and mend while taking care of the built-in mechanisms that maintain our cells healthy. Our body naturally goes through processes like autophagy to maintain the health of our cells, which keeps us healthy.

To help our body purge damaged cells and regenerate new, healthier ones, autophagy is the process our cells go through to remove waste and defective cells. According to evidence, intermittent fasting increases the frequency of this process, making our bodies work harder to eliminate any extra waste and dysfunctional cells.

Increased autophagy may help prevent a variety of illnesses, including cancer, inflammatory diseases, cardiovascular diseases, and neurological diseases.

12. Intermittent fasting may Prolong Your Life

Because of many factors, including weight loss, lowered blood pressure, and the majority of the advantages we outlined above, intermittent fasting may help us live longer while also improving the quality of our lives.

Animal studies have shown that intermittent fasting affects longevity, having positive impacts on life expectancy and markets for health, stress, metabolic response, and age-related disorders.

13. May Help Foster Balance in Fields Other Than Food

Since food is what we are restricting during intermittent fasting, that is what comes to mind first. But would a break from other aspects of our lives be beneficial?

What other things could we fast besides food as the fundamental idea of fasting is to refrain from something for a set amount of time.

We might benefit from taking a break from things like television, social media, and video games, to name a few. Doing so could improve our health and well-being.

At the end of the day, making a conscious decision to change or modify our habits can assist us in setting values- and belief-based health and wellness goals.

The advantages and disadvantages of intermittent fasting

The advantages of intermittent fasting:

Numerous health advantages of intermittent fasting have already been shown, and research is still being done on them.

Additionally, intermittent fasting may be a good fit for certain people's conception of a long-term, sustainable diet.

Here are a few advantages of intermittent fasting that might interest you if you're considering it.

1. It could help with weight loss and metabolic health

Managing one's weight and maintaining metabolic health are the two main reasons people try intermittent fasting. A measure of the body's ability to metabolize or digest energy is called metabolic health. Blood pressure, blood sugar, and blood fat levels are frequently used to measure it.

A calorie deficit occurs when your body has fewer calories than it needs to maintain its current weight. This can happen when you fast or go without eating for some time. The majority of weight loss regimens are therefore characterized by calorie restriction, such as fasting.

According to research, some forms of intermittent fasting may be just as successful at helping you lose weight as other diets that also focus on cutting back on your daily caloric intake, though they may not always be.

One sort of intermittent fasting that has been directly connected to weight loss is time-restricted eating schedules, such as the 16/8 technique. The 5:2 diet as well as alternate-day fasting might be helpful.

In addition to reducing your calorie intake during the fasting phase naturally, intermittent fasting may aid in weight loss by managing your appetite to make you feel fuller for longer while squelching hunger pangs.

2. A change in lifestyle that can be sustained

Calorie counting, eating certain meals that you might not be used to eating, or avoiding particular foods that you might otherwise love are not usually requirements of intermittent fasting.

One method of intermittent fasting, for instance, is to eat dinner early and then wake up late. You have technically fasted for 16 hours if you finish your last meal at 8 p.m. and don't eat again until noon the following day.

3. Works well with a diet rich in whole foods.

Intermittent fasting is typically simple to incorporate into your current diet because it places more emphasis on when you eat than what you consume. You won't need need to purchase any special foods or make any changes to your normal diet.

Fasting may be a viable option for you to consider if you are currently happy with the state of your food but are seeking additional ways to improve your general health.

4. Could Be Good For Heart Health

One of the most dangerous illnesses in the United States is heart disease. Your chance of developing heart disease and the risk factors that increase that risk may be reduced by intermittent fasting. You can lower your blood pressure, cholesterol, and blood sugar levels by fasting.

5. Could Benefit Your Brain

In the case of intermittent fasting, some people may be correct when they assert that what is excellent for your body is also good for your brain. Reduced stress, less inflammation, and lower blood sugar levels are just a few of the effects of fasting. All of these aid in reducing stress and promoting relaxation. The proliferation of nerve cells may be accelerated during intermittent fasting, which is advantageous for brain health.

6. Could Boost Your Immune System

Additionally, it has been shown that fasting can cause your body's old cells to regenerate, including immune system cells. Your immune system's cells can grow stronger and be better able to fend off illnesses by renewing.

As was previously mentioned, fasting can help you lose weight and flush toxins from your body, which can strengthen your immune system.

Disadvantages of Intermittent Fasting

When you initially start intermittent fasting, you can experience some of the drawbacks listed below.

1. Contrary to what you may expect.

Intermittent fasting calls for planning, restraint, and discipline.

It may not be a problem for some people to use those strategies to limit their calorie consumption to a certain period, but it may feel strange to some people at first. If you typically eat when you feel like it, this may be particularly true for you.

Furthermore, it could be difficult to stick to a certain period for your caloric intake if your schedule tends to change from day to day due to duties to your family, job, or other commitments.

You'll probably feel hungry, and if you're not used to fasting, even an 8 or 12-hour fast may seem like a long time.

Several times a week, you might go to bed hungry. Naturally, that could feel unpleasant and ultimately unsustainable. This is not to say that you can't grow used to fasting regularly.

2. **Intermittent fasting may even make you feel less hungry once you've become used to it.**

After a few months, many people become used to the routine and some even start to like it. But first, it's important to expect and be mindful of feelings of hunger and irritation.

3. Your mood may be impacted by the side effects.

In addition to feeling more hungry when you initially start intermittent fasting, mood swings are another thing you could experience. This is reasonable. Fasting can have adverse effects, such as headaches, constipation, exhaustion, sleep difficulties, and more, in addition to initially boosting hunger levels.

Furthermore, anger and anxiety are typical signs of low blood sugar. This is a typical biological reaction to calorie restriction or fasting. Your emotional health may, however, be another negative effect of intermittent fasting that will become better with time and practice. Intermittent fasting may even make you feel proud or accomplished once you've had time to adjust.

As a result, Some people, but not all, find success with intermittent fasting as a weight loss strategy.

To sum up, Some people find success with intermittent fasting as a weight loss strategy, but not everyone does.

For those who currently have or have had an eating disorder, it is not advised. Children, people with preexisting medical issues, and women who are pregnant or nursing may not be able to use it.

If you choose to experiment with intermittent fasting, keep in mind that, as with any eating strategy, diet quality is essential.

Eat a range of nutrient-dense whole meals within your eating window and avoid eating too many ultra-processed foods to get the maximum benefits from intermittent fasting.

Additionally, make sure to speak with a qualified healthcare practitioner to confirm that starting an intermittent fast is safe for you to undertake.

4. Could Encourage Binge Eating

Many people tend to overeat on "feasting" days, which are days when you are permitted to eat, as a result of the way intermittent fasting is arranged. Because there are no restrictions on meal size or frequency on these "feasting" days, some people might overeat to make up for their earlier fasting days. Your hunger may become more intense because you are depriving your body of food on specific days or at specific times. This will also cause you to overeat and make unhealthier food choices.

5. Could lessen physical activity

Fasting has the additional disadvantage of decreasing your physical activity. It is not advised that you engage in vigorous exercise while following an intermittent fasting diet. Even if you continue your normal physical activities, you could feel worn out and tired. If you're an athlete, intermittent fasting is not suggested.

6. Could exhaust and depress you

You can experience unusual levels of fatigue and irritability if you fast intermittently. Because you aren't eating enough, intermittent fasting places your body under extreme stress. This increases stress, which strains your neural system and can result in exhaustion, burnout, poor energy, low body temperature, and a decline in hormone production.

7. Might Contribute to an Eating Disorder

Another technique to deprive your body of food is intermittent fasting. It is a kind of restrictive eating that demonstrates a clear link between weight loss and completely skipping meals. You can drop more weight by skipping more calories and/or fasting for a longer period.

Fasting may cause an eating disorder relapse or even the emergence of a new eating disorder if you have previously struggled with one. Since skipping meals is encouraged by any diet, it may result in certain unfavorable interpersonal interactions. Any diet that encourages missing meals, after all, might result in some unhealthy interactions with food.

Although we've listed some possible benefits and drawbacks of intermittent fasting, because the practice is so recent, there isn't much research on it yet. Research and analyze your alternatives for yourself before determining whether intermittent fasting is right for you.

Chapter 2

Types of Intermittent Fasting

Even though not everyone who practices intermittent fasting sees these advantages, enough positive experiences (especially those posted on social media) have persuaded many people that this eating strategy is worthwhile a shot. Then you might want to look into these five different types of intermittent fasting.

1. Time-Restricted Intermittent Fasting

For those who practice time-restricted eating, this entails squeezing all of their meals and snacks into a small window of time, followed by a period of fasting for the remainder of the day.

This method of intermittent fasting is the most popular and is excellent for beginners because it only requires skipping late-night snacks and postponing breakfast for a few hours to get started. Sounds simple enough.

Additionally, during the fasting window, you are allowed to drink water, unsweetened tea, and black coffee, which may make you feel less deprived.

Another benefit is that since the majority of the fasting window falls during sleep, time-restricted programs are simple to implement into daily life. There are several approaches to this type of Intermittent Fasting:

- **16:8 Intermittent Fasting Schedule**

The 16:8 method of intermittent fasting entails limiting your daily eating window to eight hours and observing a 16-hour fast every day. This regimen typically entails foregoing breakfast and all food after dinner. You could eat, say, between midday and 8 p.m.

Have you ever heard a person who fasts claim they skip breakfast or demand an early dinner? They most likely follow the 16:8 plan, which is the most widely used schedule, which explains this. Following a 16-hour fast (often overnight and a little more), you have an 8-hour window where you can eat as many as two or three meals.

- **14:10 Intermittent Fasting Schedule**

Same as the above, but with a slightly shorter fasting period (14 hours) and longer eating window (10 hours).

It could be challenging for some people to lose weight with this diet because the fasting period is brief and closely resembles how they already eat. However, it may be beneficial.

- **12:12 Intermittent Fasting Schedule**

Many first-timers start here; by skipping evening snacks, your body will start to fast as soon as you eat supper. then have breakfast at the regular time.

Delay your breakfast every day by an hour until you've extended your fast to 14 or 16 hours to advance with this intermittent fasting technique. What about 16 hours is so special? It takes that long for your body to go from burning carbs (if you recently had any) to burning fat.

Additionally, it starts the process of autophagy, or cellular cleansing and regeneration. Reduced inflammation and potential defense against age-related diseases like Parkinson's and Alzheimer's are two examples of the health benefits attributed to autophagy.

Organizing your meals to coincide with your eating window becomes automatic once you get into the swing of things.

2. Modified-Calorie Intermittent Fasting

Modified-calorie eating plans combine time restriction with reduced calorie intake on certain days. The goal: kicking your body's fat-burning into overtime, as a lack of ready-to-burn fuel options such as carbohydrates forces it to dig deep into the reservoirs in fat cells, thus expending more energy and driving weight loss. The best-known modified calorie plan is the 5:2 method.

- **5:2 method**

The modified calorie diet in this form recommends eating normally five days a week and restricting caloric intake to roughly 500 calories for women and 600 calories for men on the two other days.

Although it is not necessary to undertake the two fasting days back-to-back, some experts feel it is more beneficial because it provides your body more time to stay fast.

The night before your first day of restricted caloric intake (or fasting), cease eating after dinner to try this type of intermittent fasting.

You have two options for your reduced-calorie day: either consume one substantial meal with 500–600 calories throughout the day or break the calories up into a few tiny snacks that pile up during the day.

The following day, repeat the process, or go back to your regular eating schedule and plan a day later in the week with the same reduced-calorie setup.

3. Alternate-Day Intermittent Fasting

Similar to the 5:2 plan, alternate-day fasting (ADF) calls for alternating between days of ordinary eating and days that allow for only as many calories as 500 for women and 600 for men. For the health advantages of fasting to take effect, your body needs a full day to recover after eating.

Follow your normal eating habits for one day as you practice alternate-day fasting, making sure to eat foods like fruits, vegetables, protein, and whole grains that are nutritious and will help you feel satisfied.

On the days you fast, you can decide whether to eat all of the calories you're allowed in one large meal or several smaller snacks.

4. OMAD (One Meal A Day)

The One Meal a Day (OMAD) diet is quite simple—and extreme. This kind of fasting allows for one meal each day to be eaten (within a one-hour window), then a 23-hour fast. Fasters are free to plan their eating window whenever it suits them best as there are no dietary constraints and you can choose what time you eat.

You are also allowed to drink water, unsweetened tea, and coffee without milk throughout the fasting window so that you can stay hydrated.

To try the OMAD plan, strive to eat roughly as many calories as are advised for your gender, height, and weight during one meal. It's also essential to incorporate a range of fruits and vegetables, whole grains, healthy fats (such as nuts, nut butter, and avocados), as well as lean proteins (like chicken, fish, or tofu) to make sure you're getting all the nutrition you need.

Since the 23-hour fast is the main objective of the OMAD, you should try to eat at roughly the same time every day. However, experts also advise occasionally changing your mealtime, particularly if it's later in the day so that your body has more time to digest the meal before you go to bed.

5. Extended Intermittent Fasting

Any eating schedule that includes a fasting window longer than 24 hours is referred to as an extended fast. Some people take these to kick-start a fasting regimen or before a big occasion, but beware: Prolonged fasting can induce dehydration and even trigger the body's survival mode, which causes it to begin storing more fat in reaction to prolonged periods of deprivation.

Only fasting for extended periods should be done under a doctor's care.

When choosing one of the various fasting strategies to follow, sustainability should be the key consideration. You're more likely to give up on your chosen eating strategy if it proves to be too challenging to maintain even after an adjustment phase. Consistency is essential in any healthy eating strategy. Focus on the strategy that, given your lifestyle, you can realistically follow to reap the benefits over the long term, rather than the one that would produce the maximum results right now.

6. Eat-stop-eat diet for intermittent fasting

This form of intermittent fasting entails a 24-hour full fast once or twice per week. For instance, you might eat dinner at 6 p.m. and then fast until 6 p.m. the following day. However, you wouldn't do this more than once or twice weekly.

Remember that going a whole day without eating might be risky in some situations and should not be done lightly. While skipping entire days of meals may seem like a good way to lose weight, it is not a long-term solution.

If you skip two full days of eating, you run a higher chance of developing specific micronutrient deficiencies the longer you do it.

7. The Warrior Diet

Most of the eating occurs at night on this diet, which is very different from the others. This diet entails eating only a few tiny meals of raw fruits and vegetables during the day and then indulging in one enormous meal at night during a 4-hour eating window.

Although there isn't any specific research on the Warrior Diet, some people may find it more practical because the fasting intervals still permit some food. It is nonetheless tighter than other types of IF because the window during which you can eat heavier items is so brief and because the diet still emphasizes paleo foods.

However, this option is not long-term sustainable, just like the eat-stop-eat diet. With this little food, it is impossible to satisfy one's nutritional demands. Your energy levels would deteriorate, and you would essentially be inviting overeating. If you choose this path, you will only cause yourself harm.

Chapter 3

How to Start Intermittent Fasting and Stick With It

Perhaps the most crucial element in a successful weight-loss journey is getting off to a solid start. Few things are as demoralizing as failing right when you start. Failure at first, however, is common since nobody finds it easy to break bad habits or form new, better ones.

Numerous advantages have been associated with intermittent fasting (IF), including improved heart health, blood sugar regulation, and fat burning. However, entering the profession might be incredibly challenging. You are after all forcing your body to go for extended periods without food!

For years, intermittent fasting has been a popular trend, with followers professing it helps them with everything from weight loss to maintaining their health. Research also supports the advantages of intermittent fasting.

Recent studies on intermittent fasting found that people who followed this kind of eating strategy lost between 1% and 8% of their starting weight.

Additionally, intermittent fasting can improve a variety of metabolic health indicators, including blood pressure and cholesterol levels, and the resulting weight loss can lower your risk of developing diseases related to being overweight, especially if you combine it with a healthy exercise routine. Of course, there is a range of options with intermittent fasting and the type you choose is ultimately up to you.

However, if you're determined to try IF to benefit from it, here are six crucial suggestions that can help you get started more easily:

1. Begin slowly

The 16:8 approach avoids having to jump right in (16 hours of fasting with an 8-hour eating window). As an example, think about the 12:12 fast, which consists of a 12-hour window for eating followed by 12 hours of fasting. For instance, if you were to observe a 12:12 fast, you would eat dinner at 8 p.m. and refrain from eating until 8 a.m. the following day.

According to studies, the weight-maintenance outcomes for fasting at 12:12 and 16:8 are initially identical. Note that improved insulin sensitivity and blood pressure over the long term does occur from fasting for longer periods. To achieve a wider fasting window, first, master the 12:12 time period.

2. Instead of aiming for perfection, be determined in your endeavors.

Leave perfectionism at the door when beginning something new and particularly tough like fasting. Make peace with the prospect that you "fail" at first because there is a very high likelihood that you will. It is impractical to strive for perfection. However, determination—the capacity to rise and try again—is a forgiving and supportive mentality that you must possess when attempting IF!

3. Your reason should be made very clear.

The purpose of your actions must be made very clear.

Choosing to practice intermittent fasting knowing that it could benefit your gut health is good.

Intermittent fasting might be challenging to maintain if you don't have a goal in mind for adhering to the eating strategy. Clarify your motivation for doing it. Some hours become quite difficult, and you could feel awful at the time. Make use of your "big why" to keep you motivated through difficult times. Improved gut health is the goal for everyone.

4. "Start your day with a late breakfast."

It's simpler to fast overnight and then delay breakfast. If you typically eat breakfast at eight in the morning, consider pushing it to nine or ten. After that, you can gradually move it to any time you choose, like 12 or 1. To prevent you from thinking about eating in the morning, it is beneficial for you to remain occupied.

5. Take more water.

Strange but true: Your body has been known to mistake hunger and thirst. That's one of the explanations why many people who practice intermittent fasting advise maintaining hydration. Drinking a lot of water is one technique that helped us curb our appetite and maintain our fast. Your objective is to consume a gallon per day

6. Find something that fits into your schedule.

This advice has probably been given to you before for everything from weight loss to skincare to cognitive health. However, if it weren't significant, it wouldn't be on the list.

Make sure you consume enough water each day (9 cups for women and 13 cups for men). It is possible to confuse hunger for boredom or thirst. Try a glass of water or a cup of hot tea first, and then see how you feel.

7. Caffeine, caffeine, caffeine!

You could experience low energy in the beginning when you first begin IF. The good news is that caffeine-rich beverages like coffee and tea are OK for intermittent fasting. Warm beverages may help you feel more satisfied, and caffeine might prevent the weariness that comes with fasting.

Hold off on the cream and sugar, though. These will undoubtedly end your fast and are mainly made up of empty calories. Try monk fruit if you have a tremendous sweet tooth. This natural, plant-based sugar substitute has no calories and has far less impact on blood glucose levels.

There have probably been rumblings about bulletproof coffee and how it might work with intermittent fasting. While it may be considered a whole other rabbit hole, you should be aware that bulletproof coffee, which is coffee mixed with MCT butter, does break your fast. Even yet, the fat in bulletproof coffee isn't the worst culprit because it affects insulin the least of all the macronutrients. Furthermore, IF and ketosis can frequently work together to enhance the possibility of weight loss. Will your fast be broken by the fat in your coffee, though? Yes, to sum it up.

8. Take care not to overindulge in snacks.

If you frequently snack or binge, you might discover that your behaviors are a reaction to your feelings. Food can provide comfort from outside stressors and problems with one's mental health. We occasionally eat just out of habit when we're bored. Be aware of your reasons for snacking, how rapidly you eat, and your level of presence when you eat. The key to breaking bad behaviors is to deal with their primary cause. Of course, when you do grab a snack, choose something healthy.

9. Maintain strong general health

The unhealthier your current habits, the more difficult issues like IF will be for you. Good eating habits, however, are much simpler to maintain when the rest of your lifestyle is taken care of. A healthy lifestyle is consistent with a healthy diet. Start by forming the following crucial behaviors for improved general wellness:

- Get the necessary amount of sleep for your age.

- For the best outcomes, go to bed early and get up early (check out our recent article on the benefits of eating breakfast before 8:30).

- Prioritize energetic and filling foods throughout mealtimes (like healthy and satisfying Mediterranean Shrimp & Farro Pilaf).

- Keep an eye on your vitamin intake.

Chapter 4

How to Manage Weight Loss With Intermittent Fasting For People Over 60

It's been proven time and time again that intermittent fasting improves general health. According to numerous research, adhering to this generally simple diet can:

- Reduce weight
- Boost your metabolism to burn more fat.
- Improve your skin's quality Improve your brain's health and cognitive abilities
- Extend longevity

The good news is that you may quickly and simply take advantage of all the advantages of intermittent fasting.

The bad news is that most adults over 60 do these 4 serious errors, which could prevent them from moving forward.

Let's examine what can occur if you attempt to begin fasting on your own, without assistance from nutritionists or a tailored intermittent fasting schedule that meets all of your requirements.

Mistake 1: Selecting the Wrong Fasting Strategy

One of the biggest errors people make when intermittent fasting is adopting a one-size-fits-all philosophy. Different people's bodies react to fasting in different ways. Your results may vary from those of others.

Finding a strategy that suits your lifestyle, schedule, and objectives is crucial for this reason. It's significant to understand that there are numerous varieties of IF plans to pick from.

You can eat whatever you want within the dining window. Furthermore, even though there are no restrictions on what you may and cannot consume, some meals are preferable to others.

Your insulin levels will rise when you consume highly processed junk food, sugary beverages, and refined carbohydrates, which will cause you to gain weight.

On the other hand, whole meals like veggies, whole grains, lean protein, and healthy fats can assist you in reducing weight and enhancing your health.

- **Why It Is A Problem**

Eating processed junk food can make intermittent fasting ineffective and cause weight gain. It can also exacerbate other health issues like diabetes, heart disease, and high blood pressure.

Furthermore, healthy foods and highly processed foods affect your body in distinct ways. Because whole foods digest more slowly than highly processed foods, they don't result in the same surge in insulin levels. Whole foods can aid in weight loss and health improvement.

- **How to fix it**

Replace the ultra-processed junk food in your diet with whole foods instead. Here are some entire, healthful things you can eat throughout your eating window:

- Vegetables
- Fruit
- Lean protein
- Almonds and seeds
- Grainy foods
- Healthy fats

You should steer clear of the following foods:

- Sweet beverages
- White bread and other refined carbohydrates
- Processed meats, such as sausage and bacon

- Junk food, such as candies, cakes, and cookies

Although intermittent fasting is fundamentally very straightforward, it's also quite simple to execute incorrectly and halt your weight reduction as a result.

There are many different fasting alternatives available online, but not all of them are suitable for everyone, especially if you're over 60.

First, there are the fundamentals. You will feel restricted if you choose a fasting regimen that departs too much from your normal eating habits and way of life. This can easily result in food cravings and overeating. When you always feel hungry and deprived of food, it's simple to lose motivation.

Then, several age-related considerations must also be taken into account.

Your metabolism is already significantly slower than it used to be when you hit 60. If you pick the incorrect fasting strategy and put too much stress on your body, it can generate high levels of cortisol (the stress hormone), which will further slow down your metabolism. This can reverse or worsen your weight loss progress.

There is a plan that works for everyone when it comes to intermittent fasting, and that is what makes it so attractive. If you adhere to a well-designed plan that seamlessly integrates into your current lifestyle, even the trickiest diet can become simpler to maintain.

Not all fasting regimens will suit your lifestyle or increase your metabolic rate. To analyze your lifestyle, eating habits, and dietary needs and to assist you in making this choice, you may want to speak with a trained dietitian.

Mistake 2: Not Taking Your Lifestyle Into Account

The easiest to maintain lifestyle modifications are the most effective. Because of this, it's crucial to take your lifestyle into account when selecting an intermittent fasting strategy.

Several facets of your lifestyle affect whether a specific fasting regimen will be effective for you:

- **Your schedule** - An 8-hour eating window every day may not be doable if you lead a busy lifestyle with limited time for meals.

- **Your dietary choices and restrictions** - Fasting plans vary in how flexible they are.

- **How many meals do you consume each day** - It can be too difficult to go on an all-day fast if you're used to eating three meals a day.

- **How active you are** - The amount of activity you engage in will determine how much energy you need and how frequently you should eat.

- **Your social life -** If your social calendar is full, it could be challenging to avoid eating out and attending social events.

- **Why it's a problem**

Choosing an intermittent fasting regimen without taking your lifestyle into account can make it very challenging to follow. If you have trouble incorporating fasting into your already hectic routine, you're more likely to cheat or quit.

- **How To Fix It**

Picking an IFP that fits your lifestyle is the greatest method to correct this error. Remember that IF is all about time-restricted eating;

therefore, any plan that enables you to consume inside a predetermined window will work.

Try the 16/8 technique or the warrior diet if you have a hectic life. If you lead a busy social life, you might find it more convenient to follow a lengthier fast, such as the 24-hour fast or the alternate-day fasting approach, once or twice a week on days when you don't have social commitments.

Mistake 3: You're unsure about what counts

The best thing about intermittent fasting is how much flexibility it gives you with your everyday diet. Your favorite foods lose their "gorge" allure because they are never forbidden, which is why people adore them so much and what makes it an efficient weight-loss strategy.

But when you do it alone, that's also where it gets a bit challenging. because it's simple to go too far with it.

You can undoubtedly indulge in your favorite foods without jeopardizing your progress. Finding a balance between eating what you enjoy and maintaining a healthy, varied diet is crucial.

And after you reach your 60s, that becomes even more crucial. Why?

As you become older, your metabolism starts to slow. Your body needs a specific amount of nutrients, such as carbohydrates, protein, and fat, as well as the vitamins, minerals, and antioxidants that go along with those foods, to function.

If it doesn't get enough, it simply won't be able to burn calories effectively and will end up storing them as fat. Simply vary your foods a little bit instead of significantly altering your diet.

YES! It is possible to enjoy your favorite foods while still reducing weight. However, if you want to see long-lasting effects, you must balance your intake of carbs, fiber, fats, and protein based on your age, physical condition, and health issues. The simplest way to do that is to locate a tailored fasting program that provides a personalized meal plan based on your requirements and tastes.

Mistake 4: Not Consuming Enough Food After Breaking Your Fast

Many people mistake IF for dieting. This contributes to the widespread notion that you should only consume a small amount of food within your dining window. This is potentially harmful in addition to being unsuccessful.

There is a significant distinction between the two in actuality. While dieting limits the kinds and amounts of food you eat, IF regulates the time you eat. Giving your body a break from digestion is the whole aim of intermittent fasting (IF).

- **Why is it a Problem**

Your body contains lean muscle beneath all the fat you're attempting to eliminate. This muscle is necessary since it helps you burn calories even while you're at rest, and you also need it to perform all of your regular tasks.

Your body begins to break down this muscle for energy when you don't eat enough on fasting days.

This can result in fatigue and muscle atrophy in addition to slowing down your metabolism.

Additionally, undereating increases your risk of binge eating later. This can negate any weight loss you've made and, in the long term, make it more difficult to follow your strategy.

- **Ways To Fix It**

Making sure you eat enough throughout your eating window is the easiest method to correct this error. How can you tell how much is sufficient?

It's a good idea to estimate your body's protein and energy requirements depending on your goals, level of activity, and personal circumstances. This will assist stop muscle loss and maintain a healthy metabolism.

2-4 meals should be eaten throughout your eating window, depending on the type of fasting you're practicing.

Various online calculators can assist you if you're unsure of how many calories you need. Utilizing the hand-size approach is an additional choice. At each meal, you should consume a portion of protein the size of your palm, a portion of vegetables the size of your fist, and a portion of carbohydrates the size of your cupped hand.

Mistake 5: Overeating after Breaking Your Fast

After a fast, hunger is normal, but overeating can quickly reverse any weight reduction you've made. When they first begin intermittent fasting, people frequently make this error.

You feel hungry because of the hormone ghrelin, which is also what causes you to become more hungry after a fast. Ghrelin surges when you overeat, making you feel hungrier than before. This may result in weight gain and a delay in progress.

Mistake 6: overeating or undereating.

Intermittent fasting, is the most typical trap that individuals fall into but is also the easiest to escape.

The formula is rather straightforward. You might easily undo some of the advantages you've earned and slow down your weight loss if you overeat. On the other side, if you don't eat enough, you risk losing muscle mass, which would slow down your metabolism in addition to making you feel hungry. Additionally, you can be hindering your capacity to burn fat if you lack metabolic muscle mass.

Maintaining an effective fasting routine requires consistency. Both the quantity and quality of the food you consume affect your health.

You don't need to monitor calories excessively, but you do need to make sure you consume enough to get through your upcoming fasting window. You're much more likely to break your fast if you're hungry because you didn't eat a complete meal. When you break your fast, your body will stop burning fat.

Since intermittent fasting is a time-based diet, most programs don't specify how much food should be consumed. Guesswork, however, leaves space for error, which increases the likelihood that you won't receive the desired outcomes. It's always advised to adhere to a carefully balanced fasting plan that securely satisfies your nutritional demands if you want to accelerate the fat reduction process.

When breaking your fast, start with a brief, wholesome meal. This will aid in preventing hunger without causing overeating. Here are some satisfying, wholesome foods you can eat to break your fast with:

- Chia seed-infused yogurt
- Vegetable or bone broth
- Grilled chicken in a tiny salad
- A green smoothie A vegetable omelet
- An array of fruit

To feel fuller faster, you can also try consuming a glass of water or herbal tea before meals.

If you're still having trouble, consider consuming more foods high in protein and fiber. These nutrients are well known for their capacity to support fullness and aid in the regulation of appetite.

After your first meal, if you still feel hungry, wait for 20 to 30 minutes before eating another. This will give your body enough time to realize that it is full.

Mistake 7: Not Drinking Enough Water

Whether or not you are fasting, water is necessary for weight loss. While fasting, drinking lots of water makes you feel fuller and less likely to experience cravings. Furthermore, a well-hydrated body performs its activities more effectively.

- **Why It's A Problem**

Dehydration can result from not drinking enough fluids, which can have a variety of negative health effects. These comprise:

- Headache
- Dizziness
- Fatigue
- Nausea
- Constipation

Dehydration might also make it more difficult to lose weight. This is because water aids in toxin removal and maintains a healthy metabolism.

- **How To Correct It**

At least 8 glasses of water should be consumed each day, especially when fasting. You can also sip on other beverages, such as herbal tea or unsweetened green tea.

Although unsweetened black coffee can be consumed in moderation, caffeine can cause dehydration. Therefore, for every cup of coffee you have, make sure you drink an additional glass of water.

Mistake 8: You Are Unintentionally Breaking Your Fast

A clean fast is not well understood by many people. Only drinking water, black coffee, and unsweetened tea qualify as a clean fast, which is what you're meant to do during your fasting window.

Given that many popular drinks include unmarked calories and carbs, it's crucial to be mindful of what you're drinking throughout your fast.

Artificial sweeteners, some of which can break your fast, are commonly included in foods that are near to zero calories or that are labeled "diet" or "zero-calorie."

- **Why it's a problem**

It is possible to break your fast and lose the advantages of intermittent fasting if you consume anything besides water, black coffee, and unsweetened tea during your fasting window. You might even give up on intermittent fasting as a result of this, which might cause you to feel frustrated and discouraged.

Additionally, several advantages of fasting, like ketosis and autophagy, only materialize after a protracted period of not eating. Therefore, if you break you are fast frequently, you might never experience these advantages.

- **How To Correct It**

If you're unsure if a beverage is permitted during your fast, look at the ingredients list. It is better to stay away from anything that contains sugar or artificial sweeteners.

Watch carefully for items that contain:

- **Sugar or sugar alcohols** – common names include sucrose, fructose, maltose, lactose, xylitol, and erythritol

- **Artificial sweeteners** – common names include aspartame, saccharin, and sucralose
- **Natural sweeteners** – common names include honey, agave nectar, and maple syrup

Mistake 9: You Aren't Working Out

Exercise is crucial if you want to reduce weight or improve your health. Your metabolism will speed up with exercise, and you'll burn more calories and have better insulin sensitivity. These are all things that help you lose weight and get healthier.

- **Why It's A Problem**

Some of the advantages of fasting are lost if you don't exercise while intermittent fasting. Exercise helps you burn calories and speed up your metabolism, both of which are essential for weight loss.

A common issue for those who fast is muscle loss. This is because your body begins to break down muscular tissue for energy when you're fasting. This may cause you to lose muscle mass and have a drop in metabolic rate.

Strength training can help avoid this and may also help you gain muscle, which can aid in long-term weight loss.

- **How To Correct It**

Intermittent fasting is not a justification for skipping workouts. In actuality, doing out while fasting can increase fat loss and enhance health.

Try to exercise for at least 30 minutes, most days of the week, at a moderate level. Walking, riding, swimming, or mild weight exercise are examples of this.

When you first start exercising:

- Start slowly, then progressively up the intensity and duration as you go.

- Plan your workouts to coincide with mealtimes. By doing this, you may make sure that you have enough energy for your workouts.

- Don't go overboard. Overtraining might negate the advantages of fasting and result in weight gain.

- Before, during, and after your workouts, drink plenty of water. Stay hydrated and steer clear of sports drinks with added sugar.

Mistake 10: You're not getting enough sleep

It's crucial to get adequate sleep for both your physical and mental well-being. It assists with hunger control in addition to helping you recover from exercise.

- **Why It's A Problem**

The hormone ghrelin is produced in greater amounts by your body when you don't get enough sleep. This hormone makes you more ravenous for high-calorie foods and boosts your appetite.

Additionally, weight gain might result from not getting enough sleep. This is due, at least in part, to the fact that it can interfere with the body's capacity to control blood sugar and insulin levels.

- **How to Fix It**

Attempt to get 7-9 hours of good sleep each night. Try some of these suggestions if you have difficulties falling asleep:

- Establish a sleep routine and follow it
- Avoid drinking alcohol and caffeine before bed.
- Regular exercise

- Keep the room calm, dark, and cool.

Mistake 11: Your lack of patience

Weight loss happens gradually. Results may not be seen for weeks or even months. This may be upsetting if you're used to getting results right away.

Even if you don't start doing IF to lose weight, most of its advantages develop with time.

- **Why It's A Problem**

It can be easy to give up when you aren't seeing the desired outcomes. Yo-yo dieting and weight gain may result from this.

Yo-yo dieting involves a cycle of weight loss and gain. It might be harmful to your health and make it more difficult to reduce weight.

Making mistakes like undereating or exercising excessively can arise from your aggravation at not seeing results quickly enough.

- **How To Correct It**

Give your body time to acclimatize, and practice patience. Keep in mind that losing weight is a gradual process and that you may not notice benefits for weeks or even months.

Pay attention to the additional advantages of IF, such as enhanced mental health, more vitality, and improved digestion.

At some time during their weight loss journey, everyone experiences a weight loss plateau.

There will be times when you'll want to abandon the plan and return to your old habits.

Your old routines no longer work, which is a surprise effect of aging. You must create new ones to honor the start of your new phase of life.

Quitting is never a good plan of action. Before giving up on fasting, you must evaluate your efforts to ensure that it produces the desired effects.

Is it possible that your fasting regimen is inappropriate for your way of life? Maybe you're not getting enough food in your diet. Have you given it enough time in reality?

You might only need to make a few minor adjustments to swiftly and easily continuously surpass new levels of fat reduction.

In conclusion, Although it's not for everyone, intermittent fasting can be a terrific strategy to reduce weight and possibly enhance your health.

When beginning intermittent fasting, people frequently make a few blunders. These include undereating, exercising excessively, and exhibiting a lack of patience.

Do your homework and consult your doctor before beginning intermittent fasting if you're considering it. Once you get going, remember to stay patient and keep your mind on the advantages. Results may not be seen right away.

Please read this:

Your body, health, and mind can all benefit from intermittent fasting in a variety of ways. There's a reason why people are calling it "transformative" and "life-altering."

However, there are countless approaches to take, and what works for one person may not be good for another. Your age, body type, lifestyle, and particular dietary requirements all play a role in choosing the best plan.

You can lose extra weight without much difficulty if you follow a carefully balanced intermittent fasting diet.

Chapter 5

Foods to Eat and avoid on an Intermittent Fasting Diet

Food to eat on an intermittent Fasting Diet

On an intermittent fasting diet, you should make sure to eat from the following food groups which are:

1. Healthy proteins

Your entire health, immune system, and ability to maintain muscle mass all depend on protein. To maintain a healthy blood sugar level and a robust metabolism, muscle is essential. Increased blood sugar, weight gain, and fragility can all be caused by a lack of muscle.

To support a healthy gut microbiome, include cultured protein foods in your diets, such as plain yogurt, kefir, buttermilk, or cottage cheese. These foods are high in probiotics.

Lean, nutritious protein sources include, for instance:
- Chicken breast.
- Plain Greek yogurt.
- Beans and legumes, like lentils.
- Fish and shellfish.
- Tofu and tempeh.
- Fruits
- Lean Meat
- Protein Powder for shakes (Dairy-free).
- Seafood
- Greek yogurt
- Salmon

- Eggs
- Ribeye steak
- Pork chops
- Chicken thighs
- Cottage cheese
- Plain yogurt
- Plain kefir
- Whey protein powder (without added sugar)
- Pea protein powder (without added sugar)
- Legumes
- Nuts and seeds

When fasting, it's vital to eat lean protein since it makes you feel fuller for longer than other foods and helps you keep or gain muscle. Some protein sources, such as red meat such as bacon, sausage, and hamburger meat, are frequently heavy in fat and include LDL cholesterol, the "bad" sort linked to an elevated risk of heart disease.

2. Vegetables

Vegetables can play a significant role in an intermittent fasting plan. According to research, a diet high in leafy greens may lower your chance of developing heart disease, Type 2 diabetes, cancer, cognitive decline, and other diseases. Most people should consume 2.5 cups of veggies per day for a 2,000-calorie diet, according to recommendations.

Including more vegetables in your diet while IF is a wise move because they are essential for good health. Vegetables also act as prebiotics because their fibers nourish the beneficial bacteria in our gut, promoting a healthier gut, a leaner physique, and optimum health.

During intermittent fasting, eat nutrient-dense vegetables like:
- Spinach
- Chard
- Arugula
- Kale
- Broccoli
- Cauliflower
- Brussel sprouts
- Cabbage
- Celery
- Asparagus
- Seaweed
- Fruits
- Carrots.
- Broccoli.

- Tomatoes.
- Cauliflower.
- Green beans.
- Cabbage.
- Collard greens.

3. Healthy Fats

For best health, one must consume healthy fat. However, a lot of individuals fear becoming obese, which is unhealthy. For cellular health, energy, hormone production, heat insulation, and organ protection, healthy fat is essential.

To metabolize fat-soluble vitamins and minerals like vitamin D, vitamin E, multivitamins, or even herbs and spices like turmeric or rosemary, the diet must include fat. These vitamins cannot be dissolved in water; they require fat.

Healthy fats may lower your chance of getting coronary heart disease, according to research.

Foods to Add:
- Avocados
- Nuts and seeds.
- Whole eggs
- Fatty fish
- Extra virgin olive oil (EVOO)
- Olive oil
- Avocado oil
- Coconut oil
- MCT oil
- Ghee
- Chia seeds
- Flaxseeds
- Fish and Seafood

4. Seafood and fish

During your feeding window, seafood of any kind is a great option. Fish like wild-caught salmon and sardines are exceptionally high in protein as well as omega-3 fatty acids, which are essential for optimum health and lower cellular inflammation.

Omega-3 fatty acids such as DHA and EPA are regarded as necessary and must be obtained from food sources. Unfortunately, many people who practice intermittent fasting lack this important nutrient, which is why supplementing would be a wise decision in this situation.

To maximize intermittent fasting, consume fish and seafood like:

- Wild-caught salmon
- Rainbow trout
- Mackerel
- Sardines
- Anchovies
- Mussels
- Oysters
- Crab
- Lobster
- Shrimp
- Veggies

5. Healthy Fruits

When on an intermittent fast, fruit can be a pleasant supply of nutrient-rich meals. However, picking fruits with low to moderate sugar content is crucial because too much fruit sugar (fructose) can lead to metabolic health problems and reverse many of the advantages of IF.

It's crucial to eat a variety of nutrient-dense foods while intermittent fasting, as with any diet plan. Vitamins, minerals, phytonutrients (nutrients found in plants), and fiber are frequently abundant in fruits and vegetables.

These nutrients, vitamins, and minerals can support intestinal health, blood sugar regulation, and cholesterol reduction. Fruits and vegetables are low in calories, which is another benefit.

For a diet of 2,000 calories per day, it is advised that most people consume roughly 2 cups of fruit per day.
Examples of good fruits to eat are:

- Apples.
- Apricots.
- Blueberries.
- Blackberries.
- Cherries.
- Peaches.
- Pears.
- Plums.
- Oranges.
- Melons.
- Strawberries
- Raspberries
- Kiwi
- Grapefruit
- Lemons
- Limes
- Avocado
- Tomato

6. Whole Grains

When it comes to heightened blood sugar response, inflammation, or gut distress, whole grains are a special kind of meal for many people, but for others, they are associated with all three of these conditions.

Grain intolerance is caused by the lectin or gluten found in grains, so cross them off your shopping list if you fall into this category. Always keep in mind to stay away from refined foods, such as white flour and wheat.

Optimum intermittent fasting is aided by whole grains that are healthy which are:
- Organic oatmeal
- Organic millet
- Organic quinoa

- Organic brown rice
- Organic black rice
- Organic wild rice (Actually a seed)
- Legumes And Beans

7. Beans and Legumes

For your meal planning when using the intermittent approach, beans, and other legumes are great options. They are true powerhouses, but they are also frequently overlooked. They are loaded with fiber, antioxidants, protein, B vitamins, and other vitamins and minerals. They support gut health, which is the root of all other aspects of health, help to balance blood sugar, ward off hunger and cravings (ideal for intermittent fasting), lower LDL cholesterol, and reduce total and bad cholesterol.

Beans and legumes are nutrient-dense foods like:

- Black Beans
- Chickpeas (garbanzo beans)
- Green beans
- Lentils
- Lima beans
- Kidney beans
- Herbs And Spices

8. Herbs and spices

In addition to being delicious, herbs and spices have a strong, anti-inflammatory effect on our health. They aid in maximizing the benefits of intermittent fasting. Almost any meal may be spiced up with any herb.

The best herbs and spices are:

- Turmeric
- Ginger
- Cinnamon
- Cloves
- Sage
- Rosemary
- Thyme
- Beverages

9. Fiber-Rich Complex Carbs

Your body's main source of energy is carbs. Protein and fat are the other two. There are several types of carbohydrates. Sugar, fiber, and starch stand out among them as the most significant.

Frequently, people blame carbs for making them acquire weight. But not all carbohydrates are the same, and they don't always make you fat. The kind and amount of carbs you consume will determine whether or not you gain weight.

Make careful to select foods that are low in sugar and high in starch and fiber.

According to study, consuming 30 grams of fiber daily may help people lose weight, control their blood sugar levels, and reduce their blood pressure.

It is not difficult to consume 30 grams of fiber each day. You can obtain them by consuming simple egg sandwiches, enchiladas with chicken and black peas, apples with peanut butter, and Mediterranean barley with chickpeas.

As they are simple to overeat when you are breaking your fast, choose your carbs carefully. Your body may surge its insulin levels as a result of eating too many carbohydrates, which might increase your desire for sweets (overindulging).

The foods on the IF list for carbohydrates include:

- **Whole grains** (protein pasta, quinoa, oats, barley)

- **Fruits** (apples, papaya, blueberries, raspberries, pears, oranges)
- **Starchy and cruciferous veggies** (Sweet potatoes, asparagus, broccoli, Bok choy, celery, tomatoes, spinach, zucchini)

- Chickpeas, beans, lentils & legumes
- Beetroots
- Quinoa
- Oats
- Brown rice
- Bananas
- Mangoes
- Kidney beans
- Avocado
- Carrots
- Brussels sprouts
- Almonds
- Chia seeds

10. Probiotics and Multivitamins

I think it's wise to keep taking your regular vitamins when fasting. I also take my multivitamins and probiotics when fasting to prevent fatigue and provide my gut with a good supply of immune-boosting probiotics. Your body lacks some of the typical nutrients you obtain from your meals when you are fasting.

Maintaining your vitamin and probiotic regimen will help you feel more energized, less headachey, and lightheaded, and give your gut a boost with healing bacteria.

11. For Hydration:

Indeed, this isn't strictly food, yet it's vital to surviving IF.

The recommended daily hydration intake is as follows:

- Men should drink about 15.5 cups (3.7 liters).

- Women should drink about 11.5 cups (2.7 liters).

Water and foods, and beverages with water are examples of fluids.

Your health is dependent on maintaining adequate hydration when intermittent fasting. Headaches, excessive fatigue, and vertigo can all be symptoms of dehydration. Dehydration can exacerbate or even seriously worsen these fasting adverse effects if you already struggle with them.

Almost all of your body's major organs depend on water for good health. Avoiding this as part of your fast would be stupid. You know, just being alive depends on your organs.

Each person has to drink a different amount of water depending on their sex, height, weight, degree of activity, and environment. However, the color of your urine is a reliable indicator. It should always be a light yellow color.

Dehydration can result in headaches, weariness, and lightheadedness, and dark yellow urine is a sign of this condition. You have a recipe for disaster or, at the very least, incredibly dark pee when you combine that with scarce food.

If the idea of drinking plain water bores you, flavor it with some lemon juice, mint leaves, or cucumber slices.

The foods to eat while intermittent fasting for hydration include:
- Water

- Sparkling water
- Black coffee or tea
- Watermelon
- Strawberries
- Cantaloupe
- Peaches
- Oranges
- Skim milk
- Lettuce
- Cucumber
- Celery
- Tomatoes
- Plain yogurt

It's interesting to note that drinking plenty of water can aid in weight loss. According to study, maintaining appropriate hydration can aid in weight loss by:

- Lowering food intake or appetite.
- Accelerating the fat burning

Here's why H2O dominates.

If you don't already have a favorite sweet water bottle, it might be time to make a purchase.

According to studies, water is the most consumed beverage in the United States. This is a positive statistic considering that carbonated soft drinks were the most popular.

Drinks with added sugar significantly increase the risk of obesity, type 2 diabetes, heart disease, and other illnesses.

You can lower your risk by drinking water instead of soda, juice, and other sugar-filled "soft drinks." Additionally, it provides several health advantages for your body, some of which you would not anticipate. Look at this.

- **Maintaining balance**

Your body is composed of 60 percent water. Maintaining your body's fluid balance helps with digestion, nutrient transportation, temperature regulation, and other processes. This is accomplished by drinking enough water.

- **Control of munch**

Water consumption may aid with weight loss. According to studies, drinking water can help you drop a few pounds. The covert motive? Simply put, drinking water makes people feel fuller and helps them eat fewer calories.

- **Fuels the muscle**

You lose water from your muscles when you sweat at the gym. And when your muscles are dehydrated, they become fatigued. Try simply filling up your water bottle and taking a few swigs to give yourself an energy boost or to help you get through that last set of squats.

- **Kidney support**

Every day, your kidneys filter away waste and transfer the urine to your bladder as they process roughly 150 quarts of blood. However, they require the proper amount of water to flush out the substances your body doesn't require.

increased productivity

You could find that a glass of water will help you concentrate at work. Even slight dehydration, according to research, can impair memory and concentration. Reliable Source

Furthermore, you'll need to use the restroom more frequently as you drink more. You'll also stay more awake thanks to those brief trips to the bathroom.

- **Energy booster**

Coffee, step aside because water can also combat weariness. Fatigue is among the most prevalent signs of dehydration. Another good excuse to take a huge gulp!

- **Help with hangovers**

If alcohol has taken its toll on you, drink a glass of water to hydrate your body and ease the headache.

- **Keep the process going**

Nobody likes having digestive problems. Drinking more water may help things, well, move along as research has shown that dehydration causes constipation in some people.

- **Fight against illness**

When you're sick, drinking water may help you feel better. However, it hasn't been scientifically established that drinking fluids can cure colds, so don't substitute this for a trip to the doctor or other cold treatments.

- **The brainwasher**

According to study, students who carry water into the test room tend to receive better grades, indicating that water encourages clearer thinking.

It doesn't hurt to give it a shot, even though it's unclear whether drinking the water had anything to do with receiving a higher grade.

Your course of action

I advise you to drink 9 to 13 glasses daily. Your requirements change according to your degree of exercise, age, and the amount of water you consume.

Foods to Avoid on an Intermittent Fasting Diet

Some meals aren't as beneficial to eat as part of an intermittent fasting plan. Foods that are high in calories, a saturated fat that is bad for your heart and salt should be avoided.

After a fast, they won't satisfy you and can even make you feel more ravenous.

Additionally, they offer little to no nutrition.

Limit the following foods to maintain a healthy intermittent eating schedule:
- Processed foods
- Sugar-sweetened beverages
- Candy bars
- Alcoholic beverages

- Snack chips.
- Pretzels and crackers.
- Calorie-dense foods or Zero Calorie foods
- Artificial Sweeteners
- Saturated and trans-fat
- Snack chips
- Ketchup
- Sugary cereals and granola
- Processed meats
- Refined grains and starches

You should also stay away from foods that include a lot of added sugar. If you're fasting intermittently, you don't want to consume sugar because it is nutritionally empty and only provides sweet empty calories. Sugar is found in processed foods and beverages. Due to how quickly the sugar metabolizes, it will make you feel hungry.

The following are some examples of sugary things you should avoid if you're fasting intermittently:

- Cookies.
- Candy.
- Cakes.
- Fruit drinks.
- Highly sweetened coffee and teas.
- Sugary cereals with little fiber and granola.

Things to Know When Combining Intermittent Fasting with Particular Diets

Some people think it's more successful to lose weight by combining IF with specific diets like the keto diet or a vegetarian diet. But whether this is true or not is still up for debate.

Do you want to combine the keto diet with IF? Include the following foods in your high-fat, low-carb diet if you plan to practice intermittent fasting:

1. **For Fats (75% of your daily calories)**
   - Avocados
   - Nuts
   - Cheese
   - Whole eggs

- Dark chocolate
- Fatty fish
- Chia seeds
- Extra virgin olive oil (EVOO)
- Full-fat yogurt

2. For Protein (20% of your daily calories)

- Poultry and fish
- Eggs
- Seafood
- Dairy products such as milk, yogurt, and cheese
- Seeds and nuts
- Beans and legumes
- Soy
- Whole grains

3. For Carbs (5% of your daily calories)

- Sweet potatoes
- Beetroots
- Quinoa
- Oats
- Brown rice

The following foods are on the vegetarian intermittent fasting food list:

1. For Protein
- Dairy products such as milk, yogurt, and cheese
- Seeds and nuts
- Beans and legumes
- Soy
- Whole grains

2. For Carbs
- Sweet potatoes

- Beetroots
- Quinoa
- Oats
- Brown rice
- Bananas
- Mangoes
- Apples
- Berries
- Kidney beans
- Pears
- Avocado
- Carrots
- Broccoli
- Brussels sprouts
- Almonds
- Chia seeds
- Chickpeas

3. For Fats

- Avocados
- Nuts
- Cheese
- Dark chocolate
- Chia seeds
- Extra virgin olive oil (EVOO)
- Full-fat yogurt

One of the strategies for healthy weight loss is intermittent fasting.

Foods like vegetables, nuts, seeds, lean proteins, and fruits can improve the effects of intermittent fasting on weight loss.

The secret to avoiding nutritional shortages while intermittent fasting is a healthy diet.

Fasting can be used with well-liked eating plans like the keto diet or a vegetarian one.

How to safely fast and shorten your fasting period

A growing number of people are adopting the eating pattern known as intermittent fasting, which entails going without meals for periods or severely limiting them.

Short-term increases in human growth hormone (HGH) and alterations in gene expression have both been connected to this fasting technique as potential health advantages.

These outcomes are related to longer life expectancy and a lower chance of illness. As a result, those who fast frequently want to get in shape or live a longer, healthier life.

But if it's not done well, fasting can be harmful.

Here are some suggestions to make fasting safer and shorter.

1. **The length of your fast is entirely up to you because there is no one right method to observe it.**

Popular routines consist of:

- The 5:2 Pattern recommends cutting calories two days a week (500 calories per day for women and 600 for men).

- The 6:1 Pattern is comparable to the 5:2, except just one day of calorie restriction is required instead of two.

- Eat, Stop, Eat A 24-hour total fast once or twice every week.

- The 16:8 Pattern entails only eating inside an eight-hour window and going without meals for 16 hours each day of the week.

The majority of these regimens recommend brief fasting windows of 8–24 hours. Although some people want to fast for 48 or even 72 hours, this is a personal choice.

Your risk of experiencing problems while fasting rises with longer fasting intervals. This includes thirst, irritability, mood swings, dizziness, hunger, low energy, and difficulty concentrating.

The best way to prevent these side effects is to stick to shorter fasting periods of up to 24 hours, especially when you're first starting.

You should seek medical supervision if you want to extend your fasting period beyond 72 hours.

Your risk of experiencing negative side effects like dehydration, lightheadedness, and fainting increases with longer fasting intervals. Keep your fasting intervals brief to lower your risk.

On days when you're fasting, only consume a small amount of food.

In general, fasting entails a temporary removal of all food and liquids.

On fast days, you can go without eating at all, although other fasting schedules, like the 5:2 diet, let you ingest up to 25% of your daily caloric needs.

If you wish to try fasting, it could be wiser to limit your caloric intake such that you only eat a modest amount of food on your fast days.

This strategy might lessen some of the dangers of fasting, like feeling weak, hungry, and distracted.

> **2. Since you'll probably feel less hungry, it may also make fasting more tenable.**

On days when you're fasting, eating a tiny bit of food rather than nothing at all may help you avoid unpleasant side effects and stave off hunger.

> **3. Keep yourself hydrated.**

It's vital to consume enough fluids when fasting because mild dehydration can cause headaches, thirst, dry mouth, and weariness.

To stay hydrated, the majority of health officials advise following the 88 rule, which calls for eight 8-ounce glasses of liquid (a little less than 2 liters in total) each day.

Although it's probably in this range, the precise amount of liquids you require will depend on many different factors.

It's extremely simple to become dehydrated while on a fast because you acquire roughly 20–30% of the fluid your body needs from eating.

Many people try to consume 8.5–13 cups (2–3 liters) of water each day while fasting. However, your thirst should let you know when you need to drink more, so pay attention to your body.

While fasting, you run the risk of being dehydrated because some of your daily fluid requirements are met by meals. Listen to your body and just drink when you are thirsty to avoid this.

4. Walk or practice meditation

It might be challenging to refrain from eating on fast days, especially if you're bored and peckish.

Keeping active is one strategy to prevent unwittingly breaking your fast.

Walking and meditation are two activities that don't need a lot of energy yet may help you avoid feeling hungry.

But any leisurely, low-intensity activity would keep your mind occupied. Read a book, take a bath, or listen to a podcast.

Your fast days may be simpler if you keep active with low-intensity activities like walking or meditation.

5. Avoid Breaking fasts without a feast

After a period of constraint, it may be tempting to indulge in a large dinner as a celebration.

But if you break your fast with a feast, you might feel bloated and exhausted.

Furthermore, feasting can hinder your long-term weight loss goals by stalling or reducing your progress.

Consuming too many calories after a fast will lower your calorie deficit because your overall calorie intake affects your weight.

The best method to break a fast is to resume regular eating habits and carry on as usual.

After a fast day, you could feel exhausted and bloated if you consume an unusually large lunch. Instead, try gradually resuming your regular eating schedule.

6. If you feel unwell, stop fasting.

You might feel a little lethargic, hungry, and irritable during fasting, but you shouldn't ever feel ill.

Consider confining your fast times to 24 hours or less and having a snack on hand in case you start to feel dizzy or nauseous to keep yourself safe, especially if you are new to fasting.

Be mindful to quit fasting as soon as you feel unwell or have concerns about your health.

The inability to do daily duties due to fatigue or weakness, as well as unanticipated feelings of sickness and discomfort, are some indicators that you should break your fast and get medical attention.

During your fast, you could feel a bit lethargic or irritated, but you should stop right away if you start to feel ill.

7. Take in Enough Protein

Many people begin fasting to reduce their weight.

You may lose muscle in addition to fat while you are in a calorie deficit, though.

Make sure you consume adequate protein on the days you eat to help reduce muscle loss while fasting.

Additionally, if you are eating short meals on fast days, having some protein may have additional advantages, such as helping you control your hunger.

According to research, eating a meal with about 30% protein calories will help you feel full longer.

To counteract some of the negative consequences of fasting, one should eat some protein on those days.

A sufficient protein intake during your fast may reduce muscle loss and control your hunger.

On days when you aren't fasting, eat a lot of whole foods.

Most people who fast aim to become healthier.

Even if fasting entails depriving yourself of food, it's also crucial to lead a healthy lifestyle even when you are not fasting.

Whole food-based diets are associated with a variety of health advantages, such as a decreased risk of cancer, heart disease, and other chronic disorders.

When you eat, make sure to choose entire foods like meat, fish, eggs, vegetables, fruits, and legumes to maintain a balanced diet.

When you aren't fasting, eating whole meals may help to maintain your health and keep you healthy while you are fasting.

8. Think about supplements

Regular fasting could cause you to miss out on important nutrients.

This is because eating fewer calories regularly makes it more difficult to meet your nutritional demands.

Those who follow weight loss programs are more likely to lack a variety of crucial minerals, including iron, calcium, and vitamin B12.

As a result, folks who frequently fast have to think about taking a multivitamin for both mental clarities and to help prevent deficiencies.

Having said that, it's always ideal to consume whole foods for your nutrition.

If you often fast and are in a calorie deficit, your risk of nutritional deficiencies may grow. Some people decide to take a multivitamin as a result.

9. Maintain a mild exercise routine

Some people discover that they can continue their regular exercise routine while fasting.

However, if you're new to fasting, it's important to keep any exercise to a low level — especially at first — so you can observe how you manage.

Walking, light yoga, soft stretching, and cleaning are some examples of low-intensity activities.

Most essential, if you find it difficult to exercise while fasting, pay attention to your body and take a break.

On fast days, many people are nevertheless able to exercise as usual. But it's advised to start slowly and assess how you feel when you first start fasting.

Chapter 6

Working out during your intermittent fasting

The practice of eating solely at specific times of the day or on specific days of the week, or intermittent fasting (IF), is known. Fasting has been shown to help some people with weight loss, among other health benefits like stabilizing blood sugar levels.

There are many different ways to fast, including alternate day fasting, our preferred option of 16:8 (fast for 16 hours a day and eat during the remaining 8 hours), or something completely different.

It seems sensible that you would want to keep a regular fitness program while fasting because exercise has its health benefits. The following six tips will help you exercise safely and productively while fasting.

1. Go slowly:

Yes, you can carry on exercising while fasting. But go slowly.

Fast workouts offer advantages. Working exercise on an empty stomach may aid in weight loss since your body will use fat and glycogen stores for energy rather than the most recent meal.

However, there is a potential that if you exercise while hungry, your body may begin utilizing muscle as fuel. That's because carbs are the primary fuel source for high-intensity activity. Therefore, performing your regular CrossFit practice while fasting or towards the conclusion of your fast may reduce the positive effects of your workout. If you're new to IF, you could also feel less motivated to work out hard.

Thus, low-intensity exercise before breaking your fast is safe, even though high-intensity weightlifting during a fast may have adverse effects. Walking, running, yoga, cycling, and light Pilates are some of the greatest aerobic exercises you may do while intermittent fasting.

2. You decide when to work out.

When you work out should depend on how you feel, the types of workouts you are planning, and your fitness goals, just like when you eat should. Remember, it's better to stick to low-intensity exercise while fasting and leave the moderate- to high-intensity sessions for windows after you've broken your fast.

Schedule weight lifting and other high-intensity exercises during your meal windows since these activities demand power and speed as well as fuel from your body. Consuming food before and after your intermittent fasting workout will enhance muscle repair and recovery in addition to improving your performance.

Exercise is best done directly after your fueling window if you can't do it during your fueling window. The most crucial rule is to not do anything if it makes you feel bad. Some people, whether or not they're doing IF, prefer to work out after a modest meal, while others find that they perform better when they're starving. Pause if you find that you are exerting yourself excessively or if you start to feel dizzy.

3. After your workout, consume protein.

During your fuelling windows, eat enough protein, high-fiber carbs, and healthy fats to maximize your fast. Within 30 minutes after your workout's conclusion, consume protein to supplement any higher-intensity training.

Work out toward the conclusion of your fasting period so you can immediately replenish if you're performing low-intensity cardio on an empty stomach. Remain loyal to foods that are entire and unprocessed and that contain both protein and carbohydrates. Our favorite post-workout feeding choice is scrambled eggs with vegetables, but if you're on the run and looking for something quick and easy, consider a protein bar or protein smoothie.

4. Water is essential.

It is crucial to drink enough water and electrolytes when fasting, especially if you're also exercising. You may have cramping, nausea, low blood pressure, low blood sugar, headaches, dizziness, and low blood pressure if your electrolytes are out of balance.

Use unsweetened coconut water, electrolyte tablets, or zero-calorie electrolyte drinks to replenish electrolytes. Sports beverages with a lot of sugar, caffeine, or other diuretics should be avoided. Make sure you are drinking enough water, getting enough potassium and sodium, and staying well-hydrated.

5. Wait until you've gotten used to a fat-burning (keto) metabolism before beginning intermittent fasting.

Avoid starting both the keto and IF diets at the same time if you wish to mix them. To allow your body enough time to acclimate to any changes or new routines, start a low-carb lifestyle before you fast. It's time to dial it back if you experience any mental haze, weakness, dizziness, weariness, burnout, injuries, nausea, or slow recovery from exercises. It might be challenging to balance exercising and intermittent fasting.

A word of caution: if the intensity is too great, additional exercise will likely make you feel even more hungry, which will make fasting more challenging.

6. Above all, pay attention to your body.

Exercise while fasting may not be advisable if you have certain medical conditions, especially those that can make you feel lightheaded, such as low blood pressure or low blood sugar.

Do what feels good to you by paying attention to your body! Stop, eat, and drink if you start to feel lethargic during your workout. Consult your doctor or other healthcare professional for advice on what is best for you before beginning IF or before including exercise in your IF program.

Chapter 7

Recipes for intermittent fasting

1. Turmeric Tofu Scramble

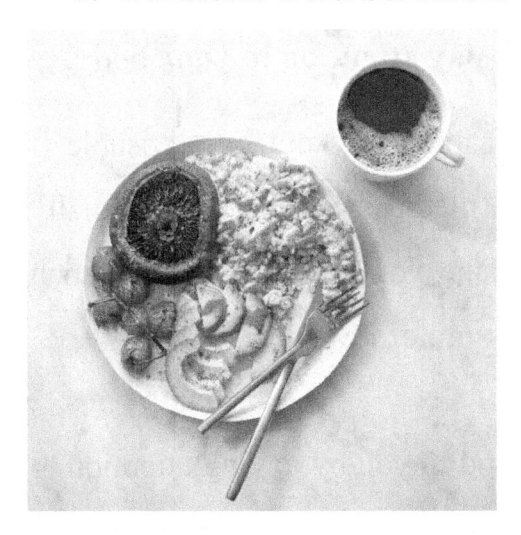

Ingredients:

- 1 Portobello mushroom
- Four or five cherry tomatoes
- 1 tablespoon olive oil plus additional for brushing
- ½ block (14-oz) robust tofu

- Add pepper and salt.
- Add some garlic powder.
- 1/4 tsp. of ground turmeric
- Thinly sliced ½ avocado

Directions:

Step 1: Set the oven to 400°F. Place the tomatoes and mushrooms on a baking sheet, and then spray them with oil. Add salt and pepper to taste. For about 10 minutes, roast until fork-tender.

Step 2: In the meantime, combine the tofu, turmeric, garlic powder, and a dash of salt in a medium bowl. With a fork, mash. 1 Tbsp of olive oil should be heated in a big skillet over medium heat. Add the tofu mixture and simmer for about 3 minutes, stirring regularly, until it becomes firm and egg-like.

Step 3: Place the tofu on a plate and top it with the avocado, tomatoes, and mushrooms.

2. Turkish Egg Breakfast

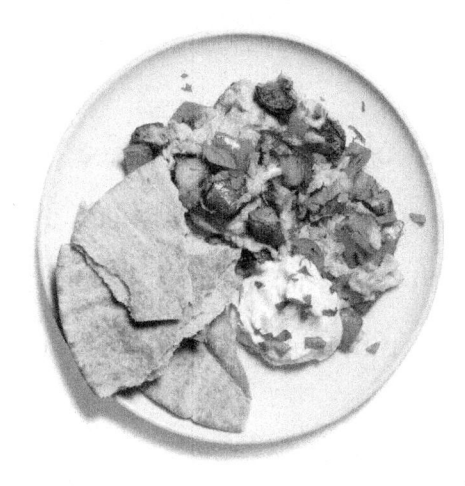

Ingredients:
- chopped red bell pepper, 3/4 cup
- Olive oil, 2 tablespoons
- ¾ cup diced eggplant
- Salt and pepper to taste, pinch each
- ¼ teaspoon of paprika, lightly mixes into 5 large eggs.

- chopped cilantro, to taste
- Plain yogurt (two dollops)
- 1 whole-wheat pita

Directions:

Step 1: Heat the olive oil in a sizable nonstick skillet over medium-high heat. Add salt, pepper, and bell pepper and eggplant. Sauté for 7 minutes or until softened.

Step 2: Add additional salt and pepper to taste and stir in the eggs and paprika. Cook the eggs until they are softly scrambled, stirring frequently.

Step 3: Add some chopped cilantro and serve with a pita and a dollop of yogurt.

3. PB&J Overnight Oats

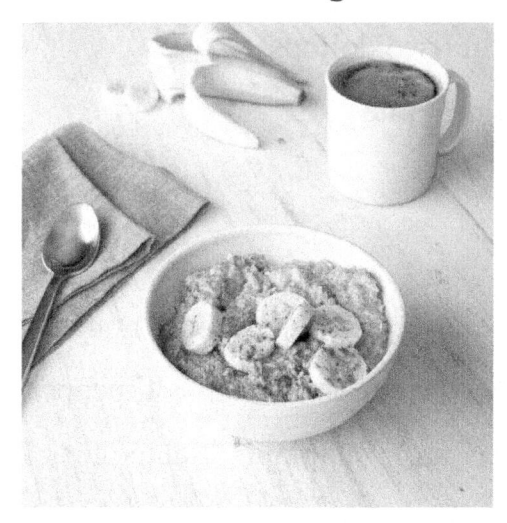

Ingredients:

- ½ cup 2 percent milk
- ¼ cup of quick-cooking rolled oats
- ¼ cup of mashed raspberries
- 3 tablespoons of creamy peanut butter
- 3 tablespoons of whole raspberries

Directions:

Step 1: Mix the oats, milk, peanut butter, and mashed raspberries in a medium bowl. Stir until uniform.

Step 2: Overnight in the refrigerator, covered. Open up in the morning, then top with entire raspberries.

4. Egg Scramble with Sweet Potatoes

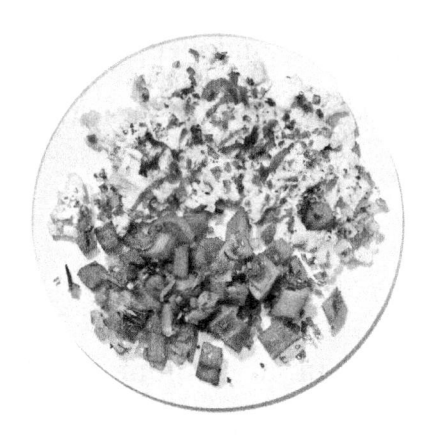

Ingredients:
- 1 (8-oz) chopped sweet potato

- 2 teaspoons of minced rosemary
- 1/2 cup of minced onion
- Pepper
- Salt
- 4 big eggs
- 2 tbsp. of chopped chive
- 4 Large egg whites

Directions:

Step 1: Set the oven to 425 °F. Toss the sweet potato, onion, rosemary, salt, and pepper on a baking sheet. Apply cooking spray and roast for 20 minutes or until fork-tender.

Step 2: In the meantime, combine the eggs, egg whites, salt, and pepper in a medium bowl. Cooking sprays the skillet and scramble the eggs for 5 minutes on medium.

Step 3: Serve the potatoes with the chives sprinkled on top.

5. Pork Tenderloin with Butternut Squash and Brussels Sprouts

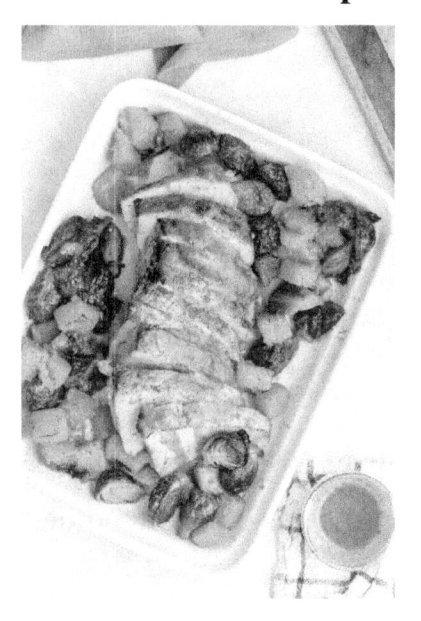

Ingredients:
- Salt

- 1 3/4 lb. Trimmed pork tenderloin
- Canola oil, 3 tablespoons
- Fresh thyme, two sprigs
- Diced butternut squash in 4 cups
- Two peeled garlic cloves
- Pepper
- 4 cups of Brussels sprouts, trimmed and halved

Directions:

Step 1: Set the oven to 400°F. Add salt and pepper to the tenderloin all over. Heat 1 tbsp oil in a sizable cast-iron pan over medium-high heat. Add the tenderloin to the shimmering oil and cook for 8 to 12 minutes, or until golden brown all over. Place on a platter.

Step 2: Then, add the remaining 2 tbsp of oil to the pan and sauté the thyme and garlic for approximately a minute, or until fragrant. Add a generous pinch of each salt and pepper, along with the butternut squash and Brussels sprouts. Cook for 4 to 6 minutes, stirring periodically until the vegetables are just starting to brown.

Step 3: After setting the vegetables on top of the tenderloin, move everything to the oven. Roast for 15 to 20 minutes, or until the veggies are fork-tender and a meat thermometer inserted into the thickest portion of the tenderloin reads 140°F.

Step 4: Carefully take the pan out of the oven while using oven mitts. Before cutting the tenderloin and serving it with the vegetables, let it five minutes to rest. As a side dish, toss greens with a balsamic vinaigrette.

6. Turkey Tacos

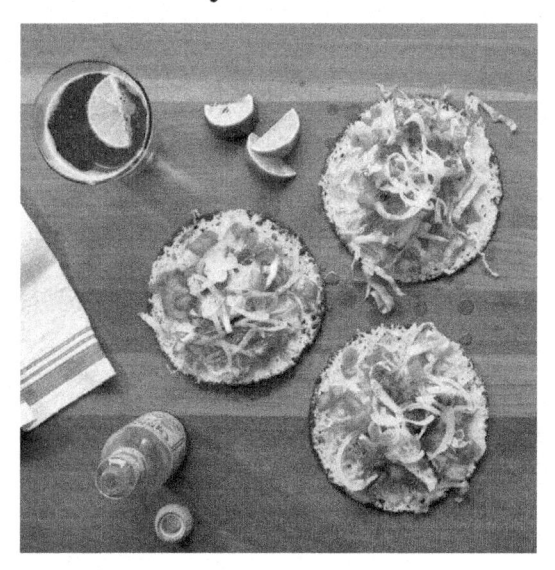

Ingredients:

- 1 cup chopped lettuce
- 1 lb. extra-lean ground turkey
- 8 whole-grain corn tortillas, warmed
- 1 avocado, sliced

- 1 small red onion, chopped
- 1 clove garlic, finely chopped
- 1 tbsp sodium-free taco seasoning
- ¼ cup sour cream
- ½ cup shredded Mexican cheese
- Salsa, for serving
- 2 tsp oil

Directions:

Step 1: Heat the oil over medium-high heat in a big skillet. After adding it, sauté the onion for 5 to 6 minutes while stirring. Add the garlic and heat for one minute.

Step 2: The turkey should be added and cooked for 5 minutes, breaking it up as you go. Water and taco spice is added. Simmer for 7 minutes, or until the liquid has been reduced by about half.

Step 3: Turkey is added to the tortillas, then sour cream, cheese, lettuce, avocado, salsa, and other ingredients are added.

7. Healthy Spaghetti Bolognese

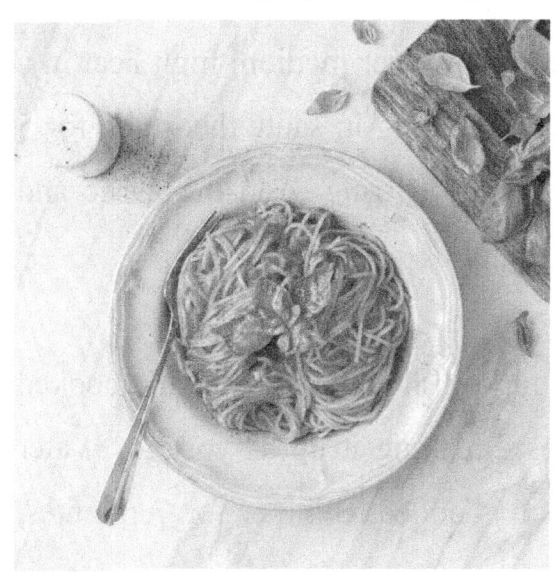

Ingredients:

- 1 substantial spaghetti squash
- 3 tablespoons of olive oil
- ½ teaspoon of garlic powder
- Kosher pepper with salt
- 1 small onion, diced finely
- 1¼ lb. Ground turkey
- 4 garlic cloves, chopped finely
- 8 ounces of sliced tiny cremini mushrooms
- 3 cups fresh tomatoes, diced (or 2 15-oz cans)
- 1 Low-sodium, sugar-free, 8-ounce can of tomato sauce
- chopped fresh basil

Directions:

Step 1: Set the oven to 400°F. Discard the spaghetti squash's seeds after cutting it in half lengthwise. Season each half with 1/4 tsp of salt, 1/4 tsp of pepper, garlic powder, and 1/2 tbsp oil. Place skin-side up on a baking sheet with a rim and roast for 35 to 40 minutes, or until tender. Allow 10 minutes for cooling.

Step 2: The remaining 2 Tbsp oil should be heated on medium-high in a big skillet. Add the onion, season with 1/4 tsp of salt and pepper, and simmer for 6 minutes, turning regularly. When browned, about 6 to 7 minutes, add the turkey and cook, breaking it up into small pieces with a spoon. After adding the garlic, sauté for one minute.

Step 3: Add the mushrooms to the other side of the pan and push the turkey mixture to the other. Cook the mushrooms for 5 minutes while occasionally stirring. Add to the turkey. Ten minutes later, add the tomatoes and tomato sauce and continue to boil.

Step 4: Scoop out the squash and place it on plates while the sauce is boiling. If desired, garnish with basil and spoon the turkey Bolognese on top.

8. Sheet Pan Steak

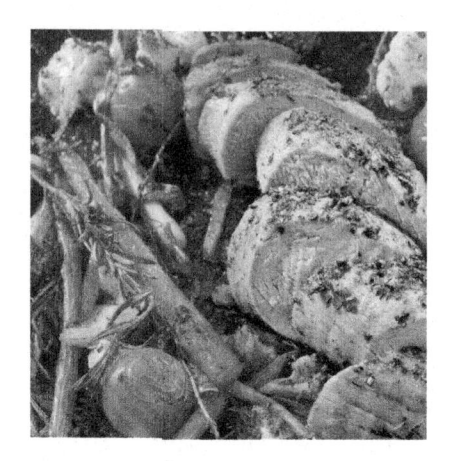

Ingredients:

- Cut and halved ib. of tiny cremini mushrooms
- Trim and cut into 2-inch lengths, 1 ¼ lb. bunch of broccolini
- 4 cloves of minced garlic
- Olive oil, 3 tablespoons
- ¼ teaspoon of Red pepper flakes (or a bit more for an extra kick)
- Kosher salt and pepper
- 2 1-inch-thick New York strip steaks, (about 1½ lb total), trimmed of excess fat

- 1 15-ounce can of low-sodium cannellini beans, nicely washed.

Directions:

Step 1: 450°F should be the oven's preheated temperature. Mix the broccolini, mushrooms, garlic, oil, red pepper flakes, and 1/4 tsp of each salt and pepper on a large-rimmed baking sheet. For 15 minutes, roast the baking sheet in the oven.

Step 2: Make room for the steaks by pushing the mixture toward the edges of the pan. Place the steaks in the middle of the pan and season with 1/4 teaspoon salt and 1/4 teaspoon pepper. The steaks should be roasted for 5 to 7 minutes per side for medium rare. After moving the steaks to a chopping board, give them five minutes to rest before slicing.

Step 3: Then, toss the beans to evenly distribute them on the baking pan. It takes around 3 minutes to roast completely. Beef should be accompanied by beans and veggies.

9. Mediterranean Chicken Farro Bowls

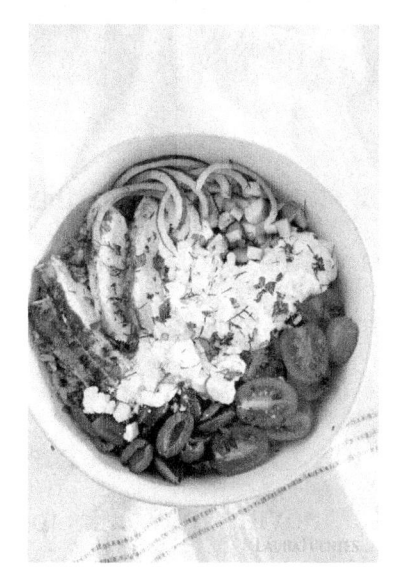

Ingredients:

For the bowl:
- A cup of farro
- 3 cups of water or stock,
- 1/2 teaspoon of salt
- 2 large boneless, skinless breasts of chicken weighing 1 pound.
- 3 teaspoons of olive oil
- Zest of 1 Lemon
- 2 teaspoons of lemon juice
- Grated garlic from 2 cloves
- Dried oregano, 1 teaspoon
- Kosher salt, 1/2 tsp.
- 1/4 tsp. black pepper
- 1 teaspoon of olive oil
- 1 pint of halved cherry tomatoes
- Chopped Cucumbers, 2 cups
- Pitted and sliced 1 cup of kalamata olives
- ½ sliced red onion

- One cup of tzatziki sauce
- ½ cup of crumbled Feta cheese
- Lemon wedges, for serving
- **Optional garnish:** fresh dill and parsley

Sauce Tzatziki

- 1 cucumber
- 1-piece of garlic
- 1 cup unsweetened yogurt
- ½ teaspoon of salt and
- ½ teaspoon of lemon juice
- Dried dill, ¼ teaspoon

Directions:

For the bowl:

Step 1: Clean and drain the farro. Salt, water or stock, and farro should all be combined in a saucepan. It should be brought to a rolling boil before being simmered for 30 minutes on medium-low heat. Any extra water should be drained.

Step 2: For the chicken: Chicken breasts, olive oil, lemon zest, lemon juice, garlic, oregano, salt, and pepper should be put in a gallon-sized zip bag either overnight or for four hours.

Step 3: Cook the chicken breasts for 7 minutes in a large skillet over medium-high heat, flip them over and cook for an additional 5 to 7 minutes, or until the internal temperature reaches 165 degrees. Discard the marinade.

Step 4: Chicken should be taken out of the pan and given 5 minutes to cool before slicing.

Step 5: Fill your bowl or meal prep container with a bed of farro before assembling the Greek bowls. Top with feta cheese, tzatziki sauce, tomatoes, cucumber, olives, and red onion. Along with lemon wedges, garnish with some parsley and dill.

Sauce for Tzatziki:

Step 1: Using a mesh strainer, line a large bowl; then, fill the sieve with a paper towel.

Step 2: Grate the cucumber and garlic clove using a cheese grater, then pour the mixture through a strainer to remove any extra liquid.

Step 3: Combine the yogurt, garlic, salt, lemon juice, dill, and chopped cucumber in a medium bowl. Before serving, give everything a last stir and chill for an hour.

10. Spiced carrot & lentil soup

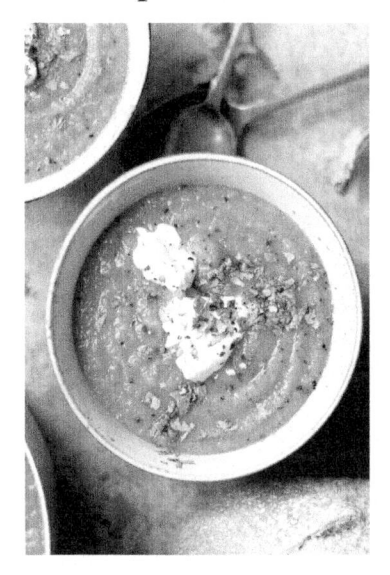

Ingredients:

- 2 teaspoons of cumin seeds
- 1 pinch of red pepper flakes
- 2/TBS of olive oil

- 600 grams of cleaned and coarsely shredded carrots (no need to peel)
- 140 grams of divided red lentils
- 1l Hot vegetable stock, from a cube is fine)
- 125ml milk (for dairy-free options)
- Naan bread and plain yogurt, to serve

Method:

Step 1: Turn on the heat to high and dry-fry 2 tablespoons cumin seeds and a pinch of red pepper flakes for 1 minute, or until they begin to leap around the pan and exude their scents.

Step 2: Use a spoon to scoop out roughly half and set it aside. 600 grams of coarsely grated carrots, 140 grams of split red lentils, 1 liter of boiling vegetable stock, and 125 milliliters of milk should all be added to the pan and brought to a boil.

Step 3: Simmer the lentils for 15 minutes, or until they have enlarged and softened.

Step 4: Process the soup in a food processor or with a stick blender until it is smooth (or leave it chunky if you prefer).

Step 5: Add salt and pepper to taste. Add a dollop of plain yogurt and a sprinkle of the saved toasted spices to finish. With hot naan flatbread, serve.

11. Sea bass with sizzled ginger, chili & spring onions

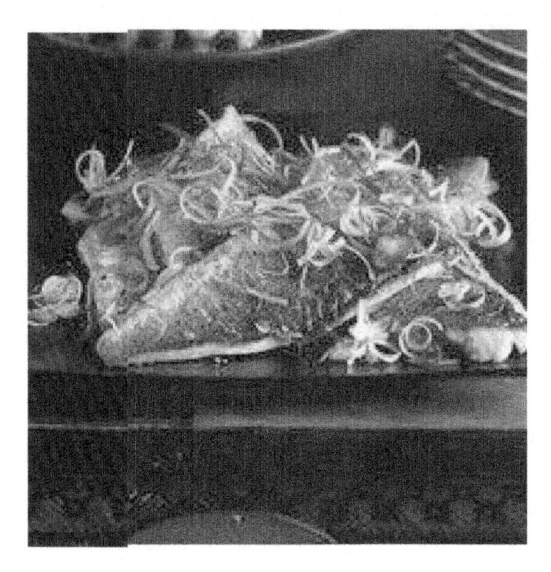

Ingredients:

- Six sea bass fillets, each weighing about 140 grams (5 ounces), with the skin on and the scales removed.
- Peeling and shredding a large knob of ginger into matchsticks
- 3 teaspoons of sunflower oil
- 3 finely sliced garlic cloves

- 3 fat, fresh red chilies that have been deseeded and a thinly shredded handful of long-stemmed spring onion
- 1 teaspoon of soy sauce

Method:

Step 1: Salt and pepper 6 sea bass fillets, then score the skin three times.

Step 2: Add 1 tablespoon of sunflower oil to a hot, heavy-bottomed frying pan.

Step 3: Once hot, cook the sea bass fillets with the skin facing down for 5 minutes, or until the skin is extremely crisp and golden. The fish will be nearly finished cooking.

Step 4: Then transfer to a serving plate and keep warm. Flip over and cook for an additional 30–1 minutes. The sea bass fillets will require two batches of frying.

Step 5: Heat 2 tablespoons of sunflower oil, then cook the large knob of peeled ginger, chopped into matchsticks, three thinly sliced garlic cloves, and three thinly shredded red chilies for about 2 minutes, or until golden.

Step 6: Turn off the heat and stir in the bundle of shredded spring onions. 1 tablespoon of soy sauce should be drizzled over the fish before adding the pan's contents.

Conclusion

Fasting intermittently may have certain advantages for the body, such as allowing the cells more time to heal themselves and lowering inflammation. A 48-hour fast is a longer fasting time, though, and not everyone should do it.

A doctor should be consulted before undertaking a 48-hour fast for anyone who works long hours or has underlying medical concerns that could make it difficult.

It is crucial to keep in mind that there are no magic solutions for losing weight.

Eating a wholesome, well-balanced diet is the greatest method to achieve and keep a healthy weight.

10 pieces of fruits and vegetables, as well as whole grains, lean proteins, and other nutrients, should be included. Exercising for 30 minutes or more each day is also advantageous.

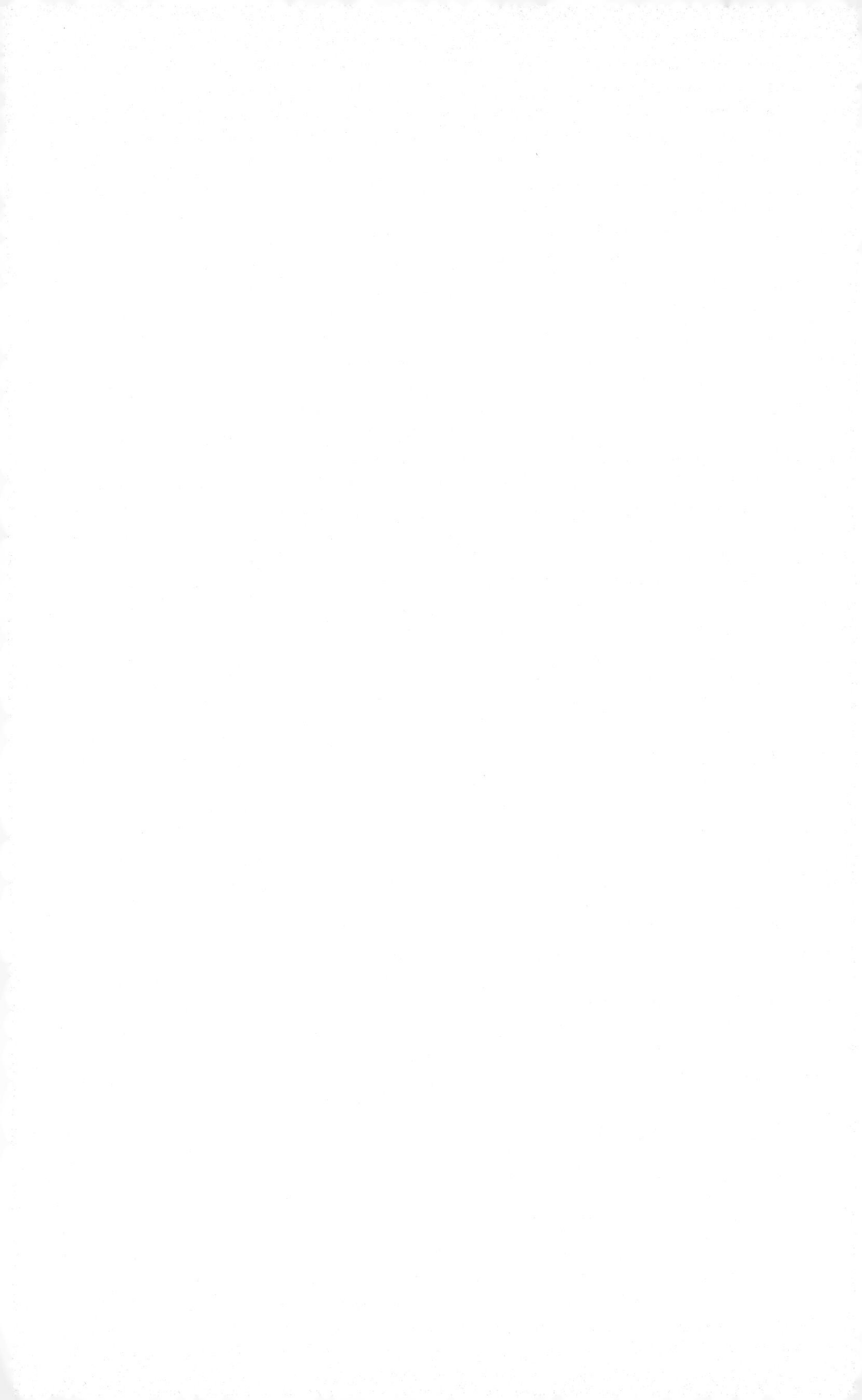

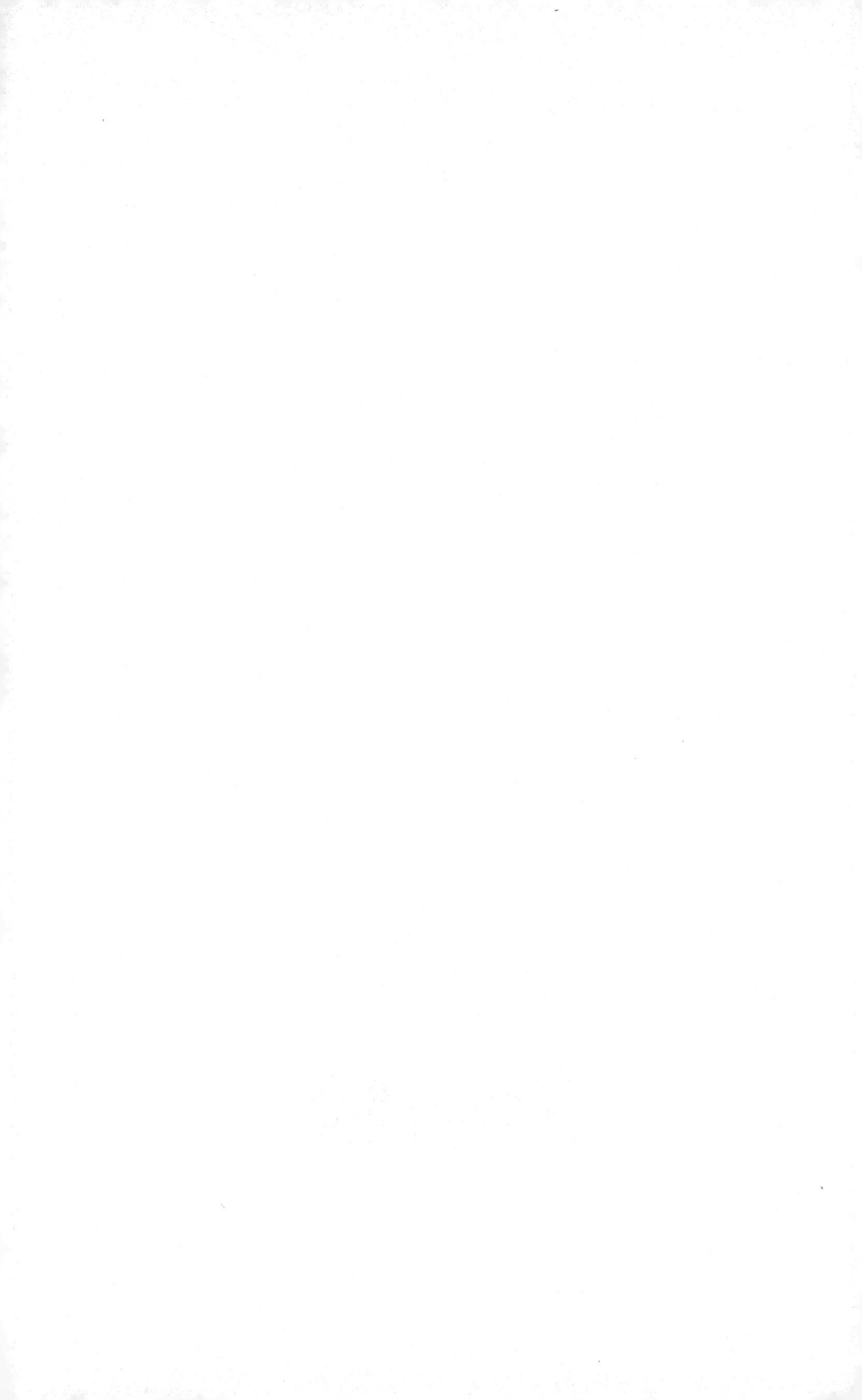

Made in the USA
Middletown, DE
02 January 2023